I have owned my dehydrator for years now and only used it once in a while. When I received Jan's book it was a wonderful revelation! She tells you, "Yes you can do this!" Her book is simple to use, straight to the point and a joy to read! Now my dehydrator is an invaluable tool in kitchen, it is in use all the time! Thank you Jan! ~

Lisa S., IL

Delicious, Delectable, and Dehydrated! is written in such a friendly and engaging style that I am not just encouraged to give dehydrating a try. I really think I can do it successfully with "Jan" at my side! The problem may be where to start!

I'm working to trim our food budget while sticking with organic produce and meats. We also need to stop wasting those expensive foods that sit just a little too long around here. After reading Delicious, Delectable, and Dehydrated! I think dehydrating will be a great tool for helping to stretch our budget by preserving the fruits (and veggies, and meats...) of the earth when I am able to catch things on sale.

Marsha W. of Oklahoma

Delicious, Delectable, and Dehydrated!

Jan Nellis

gracefarmstudios

WOODSTOCK, ILLINOIS

ISBN 978-0-9859909-0-9
90000
9 780985 990909

Jeff, Jason, Sara, Joshua, Jonathan and Jennavieve, you have always encouraged me to explore possibilities, create beauty and learn more about what excites me. Thank you for your constant love and support.

May your kitchens be humming with the joy of food preservation and your pantries overflowing with delicious goodness.

This promises to be very dry reading.

FOREWORD

It is a pleasure and honor to introduce Jan Nellis, who writes about homesteading in such an encouraging and genuine manner that even "city folk" will feel an invited guest of her cozy kitchen It is a great irony in today's world that often we must first read about the practices of previous generations in order to enjoy them. A practical guide such as this will be a treasure for generations to come.

Ann Chaney

Grace Farm Studios

Woodstock, IL

2011

Table of Contents

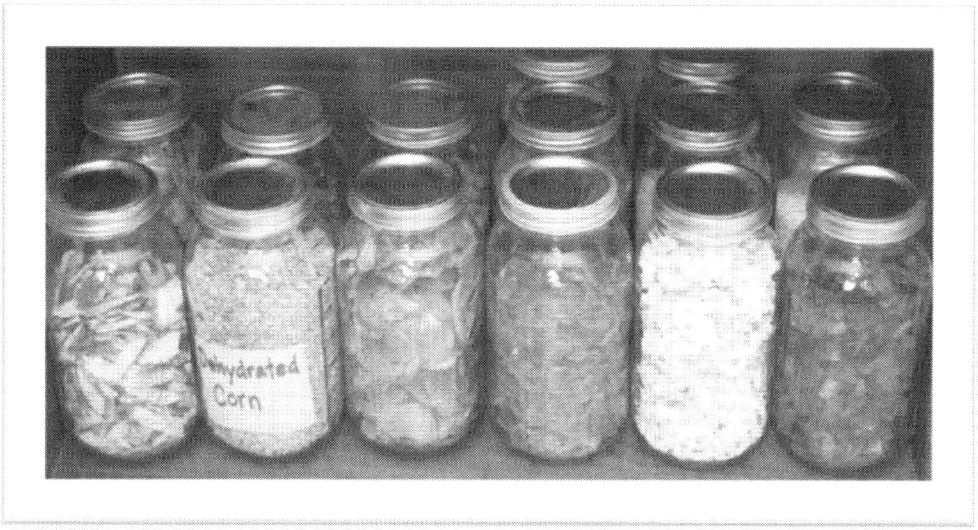

1 Why Dehydrate?

We all eat. And we'd like to have a steady supply of food around the house. We plan, choose, purchase, and store our means of nourishment. But it is more than nourishment, isn't it? We love food! We plan meals to comfort and satisfy, to celebrate family holidays, to restore health and renew energy. We enjoy sharing and exchanging culinary insight. We pass recipes across generations, coax and persuade others to share their recipe treasures, comb through libraries of recipes, and in creative moments, we even design our own recipes. All of these actions focus on food.

With so many reasons to think and plan around food, I'm forced to consider the importance of my food storage and inventory. If I learn to dehydrate, I can prepare for a rainy day, preserve harvest from the garden, create a gift from my kitchen, and store large amounts of food in a small place. I can avoid falling prey to produce laden with pesticides, fungicides, antibiotics and growth hormones. The art and satisfaction of food dehydrating helps me avoid a number of food preparation dilemmas.

My family's new-found knowledge of nourishing foods has helped us find ways to healthier eating, stronger bodies, and nutritional freedom. We buy more organically grown foods, plant more gardens, and shop at local farmer's markets. Armed with life-giving foods, we cook, eat, and serve others delightful feasts. Our freezers, refrigerators, and pantries are stocked with the ingredients that will come together to create satisfying and comforting meals. I'd like to share with you some of my joy in preserving fresh, seasonally grown food through dehydration.

As foods grow in their peak season, they flourish under ideal conditions. Nutritional values escalate and flavors are superior. This is one reason we try to eat fruits and vegetables as they are locally grown in season. It's also a great way to impact the sustainability of our community. Buying from local, organic farms also supports wise growing practices and family businesses. Neighborhood farmers benefit and continue to produce the highest-quality goods as your family becomes more dependent on what can be grown locally. You'll see your health (and the economy!) improve when you buy fresh produce from local farmers or grow it yourself. Family and friends will prosper from meals that have come from a homestead as opposed to a warehouse. There is a bountiful harvest of more than food when you delight in the offerings of the season. By dehydrating the foods you love when they're at the peak of ripeness, you're able to enjoy goodness year-round and you've purchased at the best price!

One of the tools in my arsenal of weapons against bad vittles is a dehydrator ready to use in a moment's notice. And that little dehydrator of mine rarely stops. Come summer, our faithful appliances can't keep pace with the backyard garden or bountiful offerings the local farmers have to sell. In walks the dehydrator prepared to preserve. With very little output of energy used during the drying process, requiring very little space to store, dehydrated foods sit (in some cases up to thirty years), ready to use, still packed with health-giving enzymes (if prepared with that in mind) and available at any time without requiring dependence on a constant supply of electricity.

When I purchased a dehydrator, I knew I wanted to use it for more than just a few things. A countertop of appliances unused is cumbersome to work on and guilt sets in as each contraption sits there, unused to its full potential. So I set out to learn everything I could and I've become impressed with how much can be accomplished with this rather simple machine.

Ultimately you're the boss of your own kitchen and pantry, and I hope this guide will inspire you to experiment with your own well-loved recipes. Renew, rather than replace, your favorite food options. You haven't lost a cookbook, my Dear. You've gained a method of preserving your health, nutrition, bountiful harvests, and your sanity, because providing great foods for those you love is a timely and valuable skill for better nutrition and peace-of-mind.

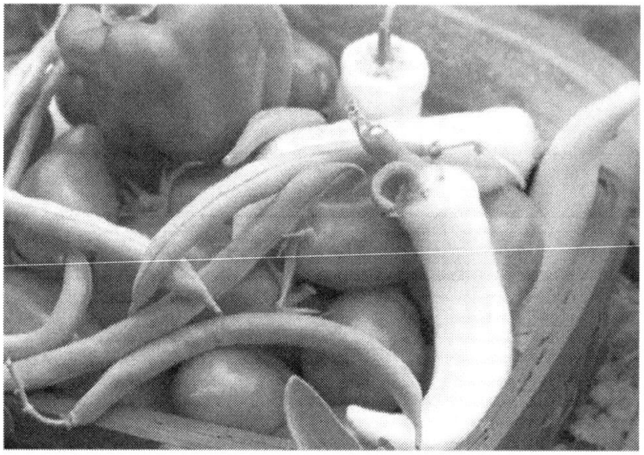

2 Getting Started

To start your drying adventure, you'll need some equipment but it need not be expensive. Feel free to purchase a new or used dehydrator. Look around a little and you're bound to find a dehydrator at a garage sale or thrift store. If you've bought a used dehydrator, simply wash it well with a 10% bleach/water solution you've made yourself.

You'll find that dehydrators are very simple pieces of equipment: a round or square container, trays, a fan, and often a thermostat and timer. Not all varieties have built-in timers. If the one you get doesn't, just set the timer on your stove, watch or clock.

What are mandatory are a good stainless steel knife and a large cutting board. You may choose to have a mandolin slicer as well since they cut uniform slices. Plan to use extreme care with a mandolin. The pro and con of such a slicer is the same: speed! You'll cut fast and be happy until you've cut yourself. Be careful.

When dehydrating, you'll need to cut all foods uniformly. When foods are cut evenly they dry equally. Unevenly cut foods will be dryer in thinner sections and not as dry in thicker sections. Your aim is to have completely dry foods since moisture spells disaster.

Some companies sell non-stick sheets to be used when making fruit leathers. The purpose of these is to prevent soft foods from falling through the plastic trays. They can be used when making fruit treats but I

Necessary Equipment

- ☑ dehydrator
- ☑ stainless steel knife
- ☑ large cutting board
- ☑ parchment paper
- ☑ stainless steel cooking pots
- ☑ colander
- ☑ steamer
- ☑ potato peeler
- ☑ blender or food
- ☑ processor
- ☑ canning jars
- ☑ labels
- ☑ food-grade buckets

Optional equipment

- ☑ Jerky gun
- ☑ Mylar bags and bag sealer
- ☑ oxygen packets
- ☑ mandolin slicer
- ☑ salad spinner

also like using them when I've pureed a fruit or vegetable like sweet potatoes, squash or tomatoes. If the puree isn't too wet, the food will dry adequately on the regular trays but can also adhere to them so tightly that pulling it off becomes quite difficult and time-consuming. If you find the company-designed sheets too expensive, buy parchment paper from the grocery store. (Parchment paper always makes me feel a little gourmet...so I've just upped the fun-factor on the cheap!)

Another useful but optional piece of equipment is a salad-spinner. These are helpful when drying cabbage, kale, spinach, herbs, or any other delicate items. Removing excess water before loading the dehydrator cuts your drying time. Eliminating moisture is the whole idea so why not give the process a jump-start?

I use my regular stainless steel cooking pots, colander, a steamer, and a good quality potato peeler for food preparation. Kitchen scissors come in handy for cutting small or fragile things. And a blender or food processor is what you'll use when making fruit leathers, baby foods or pureed foods.

If you think you'd like to make your own jerky, you may want to purchase a jerky gun, which lets you use lean ground meats. A gun may seem like a hefty additional expense but it will allow you to make jerky using much less expensive cuts of meat. No matter what you use, be aware: all meats must me lean!

And finally, if you enjoy yogurt, stop buying it and start making it. I buy half-pint and pint canning jars to use for yogurt. If you have a dehydrator that allows you to remove trays with room to put the jars, they'll go straight from the "drying" process to the fridge and be ready for you at a moment's notice.

Don't make the mistake of planning your dehydration project through to the point of dried foods without considering how you plan to store it afterward. Intend to have good quality, air-tight containers. I prefer canning jars for frequently used items and Mylar bags for long-term storage. The bags will need to be sealed with a food-sealer. I also purchase oxygen packets which get added to my containers insuring extra safety against spoilage. Five or six-gallon food-grade buckets are good for storing the Mylar bags. They'll seal with air-tight lids which need to be pried off or screwed off, depending on the lids you choose. I have both. These are especially good when planning for long-term storage needs.

Labels are good to have on your foods as well. You may decide to write the name and date on a Mylar bag using a permanent marker but you'll want to label your canning jars differently. Most foods are distinguishable by sight but some aren't. When powders are made from dried foods, you may be left guessing. The labels should clearly list the contents and date you dehydrated the food.

Begin the adventure of preserving your foods in their dried state….in a suspended state of goodness…and you'll find yourself storing a powerhouse of possibilities. Begin today enjoying foods which are delicious, delectable and dehydrated!

Drying Times

Drying times are always listed with large windows. The reason for this is because times vary based on several things. The thickness of your slices, the juiciness of the fruits, the humidity of one particular day, how well you dried the food before placing it on racks, these and similar other reasons will affect your final drying time. Even when you process your foods exactly the same way each time, the drying period may be different. Become comfortable looking at the foods, touching them and examining them for moisture. Bend, break or tear the foods to see whether they have fully dried. Under no circumstance do you want to see your hard work and good food go down the drain or to Compost Heaven ahead of schedule.

Dehydrated. . . But Still Raw

Eating raw foods has great advantages. People are beginning to recognize the health benefits of eating their foods with as little processing as possible. Many are eating raw to help heal their bodies of disease.

You can dehydrate food in its raw state if you do not use temperatures higher than 115 degrees. The drying times will need to be longer and you'll have to check the food periodically to determine whether it is fully dry but the advantages to eating raw foods are worth it.

Don't put the planning and effort into this project though if you intend on blanching the food before drying it. You'll have killed the enzymes in the boiling water before they ever get to the drying stage. And only prepare the foods to be enjoyed raw if you don't intend to cook them after they're dry.

I always dry our apples at 115 degrees so we can have raw apple snacks. If I put those same apples into a pie or German pancake, I'll still enjoy the wonderful apples even though they're no longer raw. All of the fruits can be made to enjoy raw and many of the veggies as well. I'll list the temperatures for drying fruits and veggies throughout the book at 130 degrees, but consider drying at 115 degrees for the raw value.

A Word about Organics

We're about to delve into the processes of dehydrating a wide variety of foods. Since the idea is to preserve the goodness of food and not the spray-on toxins, how do you decide which ones to purchase from the organic section of the store or farm?

When foods are peeled, you're exposed to fewer of the detrimental aspects of pesticides and fungicides. However, when you eat the whole food, it is a perfect time to consider organic. Some of the foods we eat are becoming more and more riddled with toxins that were never meant for our bodies.

I can't speak about food and not mention quality ingredients. No need to feel the pressure of purchasing all organics if you can't afford them. If your budget demands that you select only a few, plan to get the ones which will impact you the most. Berries are sprayed and we eat the whole thing. No one peels a raspberry or strawberry. Pop a luscious blueberry in your mouth and you'll want to savor the flavor not ponder the pest control used to grow this tasty treat. A cherry, grape or peach is a thing of beauty and must be enjoyed in its fullness which does not include torment about the chemicals used to grow it, The current top-ten list to purchase organically:

Berries
Leafy vegetables
Peppers
Apples
Bananas
Celery
Potatoes
Green beans
Grapes
Peaches

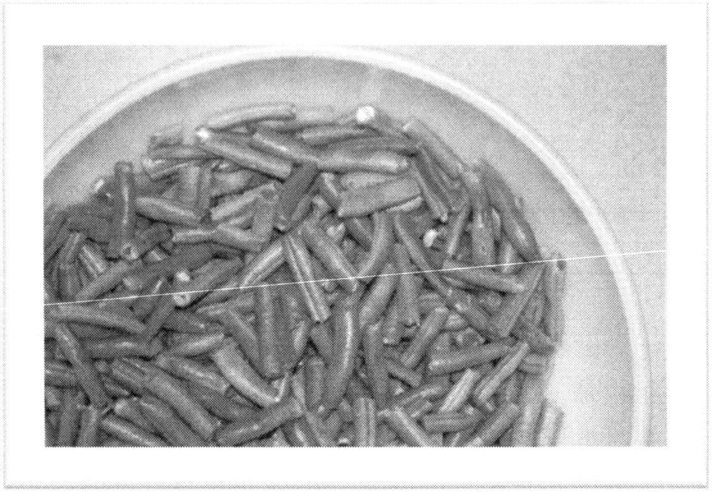

3 Vegetables

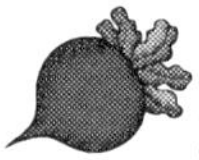

Beets

Beet salad with red beans and rice was a staple at my house on Mondays in New Orleans. I don't often hear about people eating too many beets these days but I recently read an article about dying Easter eggs using beet powder! Since I'm a spinner, I think the beet powder or juice left after cooking the beets would be a great way to dye wool. Beets dry to the deepest purplish-black with lovely concentric circles.

To prepare beets, leave three to four inches of the stems on them and cook in boiling water for thirty minutes. Let them cool slightly since you'll need to trim the stems and gently peel them. The outer skin will just slip off as you rub the surface. Chop or slice the beets ¼" thick and dry at 130 degrees for approximately twelve hours. As with all foods, store in an air-tight container.

A cautionary word about handling beets: wear gloves or expect your hands to be stained. Personally, I loved the experience. My stained hands didn't last long and they reminded me that I'd been working with the fruit of the earth (in this case, vegetables of the earth).

Beets are known for adding an earthy flavor to foods. They can be rehydrated and prepared as desired or pulverized and used creatively. Sprinkle the powder on salads or use in salad dressings. Add sparingly to soups. Be prepared for the color they'll add. You won't be sneaking beets by too many people. And if you've not tried beets because you're not a fan of borscht, look around for a few other recipes. You might surprise yourself with a new-found friend.

Carrots

Rehydrated carrots taste wonderful in beef stew or a pot of vegetable soup. But . . . Oh my! What's a body to do with critters in her garden?!

Dear Mr. Bunny,

Can I call you Bugs? *I was thinking about you this morning. Carrots are on sale again and I found a farmer with nice organic produce.*

I've kept quiet *about your little secret for a long time but something occurred to me today. What if you gave up your life-of-crime? You know what I'm talking about. You'd free up your evenings if you stopped hopping all over town rooting through one garden after another. And I'd like to see you be able to hold your head up in public again. Those long ears of yours are so cute!*

What if I can show you how to dehydrate carrots*? You buy them on sale (wouldn't Farmer Brown rather see a little cash instead of your cute cotton tail movin' at top speeds?), bring 'em over here and we'll keep you in carrots for the rest of the year. They're amazingly easy to dry and between you and me, girl bunnies like boy bunnies who can cook!*

Here's what you do: *peel the carrots unless they're organic and then you need only scrub them well and cut them up into ¼" slices. Blanch for three minutes and cool in a bowl of water. After they've had a chance to cool, place them on the racks and dry at 130 degrees for six to eight hours. If you want your slices thinner, blanch for one minute. Baby carrots dry perfectly too. Just blanch them for three to four minutes and dry for eight to ten hours. The carrots are dry when they feel crispy.*

And just so you know, *parsnips can be dried like carrots. Same exact directions. I know what a party animal you are. Live it up with a little variety!*

Gee, Bugs. *I'd do just about anything to keep you out of the slammer!*

Yours truly,

Mrs. Brown***.....Farmer Brown's wife****!*

Cream of Broccoli Soup

3 T. butter
2 cups of dried broccoli
½ cup dried sliced carrots
¼ cup dried celery
1 ½ T. dried onions
1 t. dried green bell peppers
1 ½ t. dried garlic powder
5 cups chicken broth
3 T. butter
3 T. flour
3 cups milk
1 cup grated Monterey jack cheese

Rehydrate the broccoli in 4 cups of hot water. Rehydrate the carrots, celery, onions and bell peppers in 1 cup of hot water. Let the rehydrating veggies sit for fifteen to twenty minutes. Once dehydrated, add the drained carrots, onions and celery to a pot with 3 T. melted butter and sautē for 5 minutes. Next add the drained broccoli and chicken broth to the simmered vegetables and cook for fifteen minutes. With an immersion blender (or transferred to a food processor), blend the broccoli mix until smooth.

In another pot make a roux by melt the remaining 3 T. butter and slowly adding the flour. Cook over a low heat for five to ten minutes. Slowly add the milk to the roux mixing with a whisk to fully blend. Continue stirring until thick and bubbly. Add the roux to the broccoli and heat thoroughly. Add cheese and stir to melt. Top with grated cheese and finely chopped fresh tomatoes. Serves six.

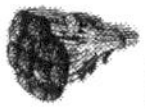

Broccoli

When given the choice between fresh and dried broccoli, I pick fresh every time. But when I'm adding cooked broccoli to soups or casseroles I'm left wondering: what difference does it make anyway? If I intend to cook it, why not have some dried broccoli in my stash?

Break apart the broccoli into approximate 1" flowers and blanch for two minutes. Put them in cold water to cool. Dry the broccoli in a salad spinner and place on drying trays. Dry at 130 degrees for six to eight hours. Broccoli is dry when it is brittle and there is no evidence of moisture.

Cauliflower

Like Dr. Jekyll and Mr. Hyde, cauliflower makes a substantial change in appearance as it goes from raw to dehydrated. The white flower quickly fades and turns brown as it dries. Your once white clusters become shriveled, light-brown masses (I know, not very appetizing). But don't worry; they gladly brighten back up once rehydrated.

I enjoy cauliflower in soups. It can be added dry to the soup if a little additional water is added. Or you can rehydrate it in boiling water before adding it to the pot. Most people today have heard about the famous cauliflower "mashed potatoes." Made similar to standard mashed potatoes, cauliflower is cooked instead and eventually blended until smooth to make a mock potato dish. Save yourself the trouble and after dehydrating some of the cauliflower, pulverize it and store it to be used as the "potato" ingredient when you're ready. Rehydrate with water and proceed with the recipe.

Cut up the washed cauliflower into small sections and blanch for three to four minutes in boiling water. Quickly drop them into cold water and let them cool. Pat dry and place on the drying racks. Dehydrate for eight to ten hours at 130 degrees. Store in an air-tight container.

Corn

If you decide to dry corn you'll find you have the makings for your own cornmeal as well as any rehydrated corn dish. You can dehydrate fresh corn or frozen corn. Make space in your freezer by drying some of your veggies. Corn is an easy one.

I prefer to use my dried corn in stews, soups or milled for cornmeal recipes. Homemade cornbread from home-milled cornmeal is easily the best cornbread I've ever eaten. And cornbread topped with homemade butter and honey sends it (and you!) right over the top. Eat some and you'll hear the angels singing.

If you're fortunate enough to get fresh corn (and don't bother with the GMO varieties), boil the corn for four to five minutes first. Cut it off the cob and place on the tray. If you're using bags of frozen corn, it will be ready for the tray straight from the bag. Dehydrate the corn at 130 degrees for ten to twelve hours. I generally stir the batch midway through the cycle. The dried corn will be shriveled and hard.

Green Beans

Leather is back in style in my kitchen....leather britches, that is. Getting their name from a southern tradition of hanging the britches out to dry, green beans resemble little pants hanging on a line when dried without a dehydrator. If you're hankering to step back in time, grab yourself a mess of green beans, a needle and some quilting thread. Wash the beans, snap off the stem end and unzip the bean. Sew those soon-to-be britches onto your little clothesline of quilting thread (about two to three feet long) and hang them up to dry. It will take a lot longer to dry than even your thickest pair of jeans but you'll have a conversational piece guaranteed to garner attention.

If you bought a nice dehydrator and plan to use it for those green beans, prep them by washing, snapping and unzipping them, then blanching in boiling water for two minutes and finally cooling them in a bowl of ice water. Lay on trays and dry at 130 degrees for ten to twelve hours. Don't be tempted to put these britches in your closet. Store them in an air-tight jar and cook up a mess of 'em when you have a yearnin' for a taste of summer.

The Culinary Trinity: Onions, Bell Peppers, and Celery

Many foods contain this great trinity. As a base for great sauces, roux or as a general flavoring, the onion, bell pepper and celery add depth and richness to anything they touch.

Onions

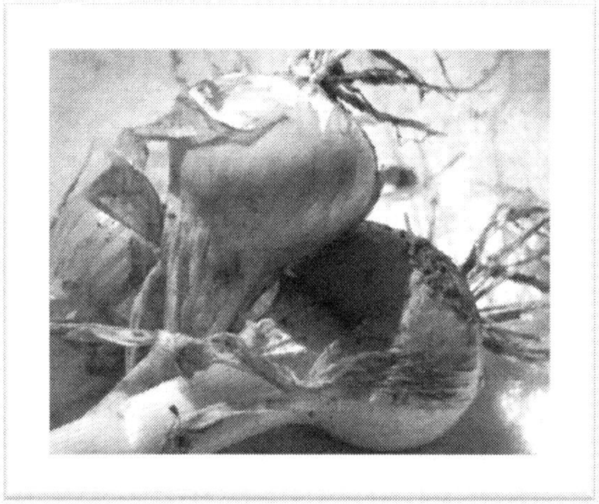

Onions are wonderfully useful and handy to have in dehydrated form. I always smile as I recall the first time I dried onions. After preparing a large batch, I set the thermostat and timer and went to bed. Overnight the dehydrating ran hour upon hour and our house smelled faintly of onions when we awoke. --- Oh, if it were only so! Our house smelled decidedly like an onion farm…only indoors. Honestly, I thought it was wonderful although no one else shared that opinion. My family begged me not to dry onions inside the house ever again. After discussing it amongst themselves, they quickly changed the begging to a simple demand. Onions were to be dried outdoors! So consider yourselves warned: onions smell strong, even when dehydrating. Did it stop me? Slow me down? Never! Onions are too useful and easy to dehydrate. You always have the option of drying odiferous foods in a garage or enclosed porch…to keep the peace in the family.

You can slice or chop the onions depending on how you choose to use them. You can also pulverize them after drying to make your own onion powder. Chances are good you have many forms of dehydrated onions in your home already. Why not create your own onion soup mix, onion-powder and personally designed herb blends?

If you want slices, after removing the skin, slice ¼" thick. Separate the rings and place on racks. Smaller rings can be put inside of larger ones to save space. Overlapping the rings will increase necessary drying time. If you chop onions (my personal favorite), keep the slices between ¼" and ½" cubed. I prefer chopped onions since they're so versatile.

Dry onions at 130 degrees for approximately eight hours. You'll know they are done when it is obvious they have no moisture left in them. They will be crispy and brittle. Drying time always varies since humidity affects how quickly things dry. You can pull trays out and stir them around. This assures the warmed air is reaching all of the cut sides. Be sure to check them periodically and store in an air-tight jar or bag if you're drying larger quantities.

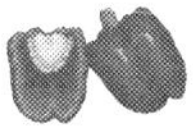

Peppers

Another great staple among your supplies are peppers…any variety will do. The culinary trinity refers to bell peppers but dehydrating is the same whether spicy or sweet. Enjoy all the choices available. Some of our favorites are banana, jalapeno and cayenne peppers. Your garden or your neighbor's might be teeming with peppers. What are you to do with such an abundant supply? Dehydrate, of course!

Wash and slice peppers ¼" thick. When I'm cutting up bell peppers (green, red or yellow), I slice half and chop the other half. That way I end up with a useful mix for cooking. When working with hot peppers, use gloves and wash your hands thoroughly after handling them.

Use the rings you've dried in a pot of chili or rehydrate and add to pizza. I always dry the cayenne peppers I get from our garden and grind them into a powder to use in my cooking. The health benefits of peppers are numerous.

Some dehydrated foods change their appearance drastically during the drying process but peppers don't change much except for normal shrinkage. The beautiful colors of the dried peppers warm your kitchen as much as the spice of the peppers warms your meals.

Wash and slice bell peppers ¼" thick then remove the seeds and place on a drying rack. With spicy peppers that I intend to pulverize, I often leave the seeds to dry with the flesh of the pepper since they add heat to the powder. If you'd like to remove the seeds to cool down the mix, do so! Dry at 130 degrees for twelve to eighteen hours. The peppers shouldn't have any sign of moisture when completely dried. If you want to use as a powder, place the peppers in a blender or food processor and pulse until completed. Store in an air-tight jar.

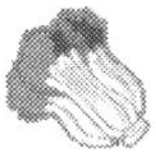

Celery

I love having dried celery on hand. Easy to buy, inexpensive and available year-round, celery is a great food to dry. Added to soups and stews, it rehydrates perfectly while cooking.

I've found myself composting celery that was purchased with good intentions and forgotten. (At least it ended up in Compost Heaven.) I've also had whole celery freeze and convinced it is no longer useful, I've thrown it out. But I hate waste. Now days, if a package of celery should freeze, I'm not the least upset. I simply prep it for drying and add to my stash. I need only run out and buy more if I'm planning to eat raw celery.

Wash and cut into ¼" slices. Blanch celery in a pot of boiling water for one minute then immediately put the celery into a bowl of cold water. Drain well and add to the drying trays. Since celery shrinks as it dries, you may want to put a sheet of parchment paper (or a non-stick sheet) under the celery so it doesn't fall through the racks. Set the temperature on your dehydrator to 130 degrees and dry for four to eight hours. Check periodically for crispness.

After drying, celery can be ground into powder and used as a salt-substitute since it has a high-sodium content. Plan to use it when making designer spices.

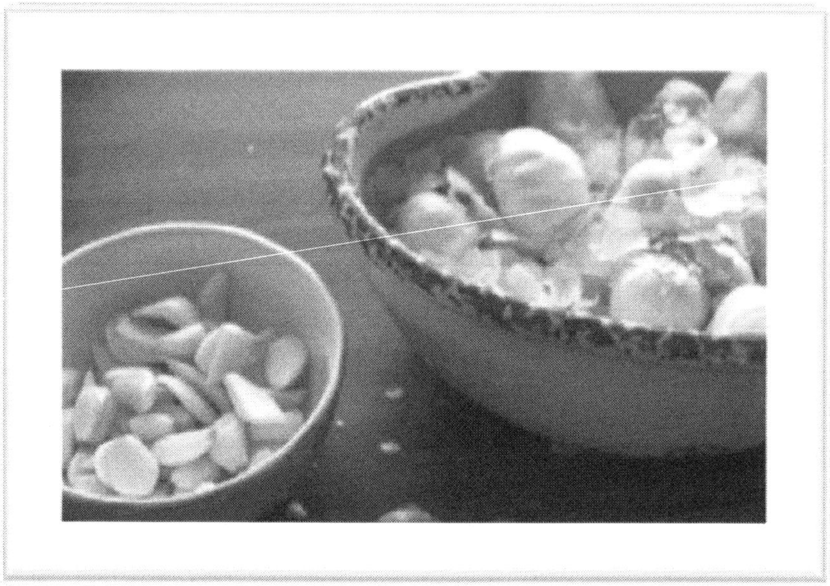

. . . and Garlic!

How long have you loved garlic? Do you remember when you first discovered it was good for you? Isn't it great when the healthy is also tasty? Garlic lowers blood pressure, is good for the heart and tastes delicious.

You may be fortunate enough to have garlic in your garden. Or maybe you buy it at the local farmer's market. If neither is available, you can purchase large quantities at the "membership stores."

Buying garlic in bulk is my preference since I use a lot, want to process it in mass due to the aroma-factor and since I enjoy making my own spice-blends which frequently call for garlic.

Set aside a bit of time to peel the garlic or opt out of the extra work and buy already peeled garlic.

Slice the garlic ¼" thick and place on trays without overlapping. Dry for eight to twelve hours at 130 degrees. Garlic will be brittle when completely dried. Store in an air-tight container.

For best flavor, store the dried slices instead of powder. Then pulverize a few slices to add while cooking. The flavor will be richer if ground just before using. As a great fan of garlic, I'm not trying to diminish the yum-factor of fresh but almost all spice-cabinets have garlic powder in them. Why not let your garlic powder be your own creation?

Leafy Vegetables

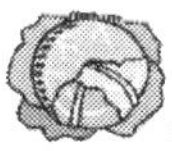

Cabbage

I grew up eating cabbage on a regular basis. In fact, I consider cabbage a comfort food. You'll find it in my garden in the summer and in various dishes throughout the year. Our home is routinely stocked with dried cabbage for soups and stews and though you won't want to dry it, we always have authentic, fermented sauerkraut on hand too.

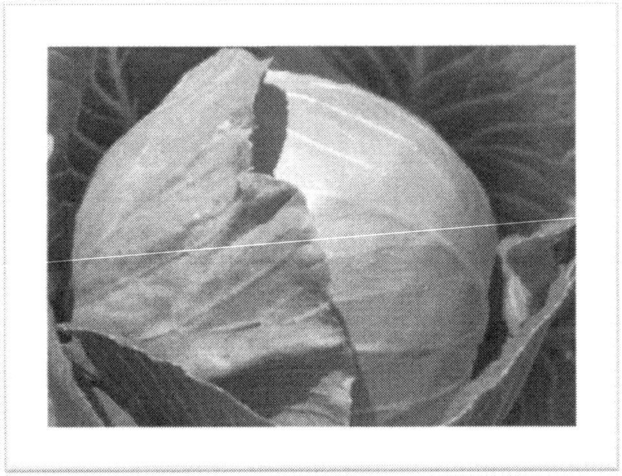

Wondering how to make the best use of dried cabbage? I like to throw a few leaves into soups. Since the leaves are so brittle when dry, you can break or tear them to the size you desire. I store cabbage in a half-gallon jar but you can always put it in a smaller jar if you pulverize it first. And chances are your cookbooks aren't teaming with recipes for cabbage powder. Just use it as you would any other veggie powder...add to a hearty stew or soup.

Buy (or grow) a beautiful head of cabbage. Core it and slice it into sections. Don't cut the pieces as though you were making cole slaw. They'll be too small since they shrink when drying. Separate the layers and steam-blanch them for two minutes. Cool and place on the drying racks. The dehydrator quickly fills since a cabbage has many layers. You may also find it easier to load the dehydrator after removing every other tray. Dry at 110 degrees for six hours. I suggest using a lower temperature for leafy vegetables since they can be delicate and more likely to burn. If you lower the temperature on any drying project and decide that moisture still exists just put it back to dry a little longer. The object is to have a completely dried food, not a recipe to follow to the letter of the law. Remember who the boss is....YOU!

Kale

Kale is another easy-to-grow food from your garden. It takes abuse and continues to flourish. There's a lot of talk about kale chips so why not make some? Or dehydrate the leaves and use kale in powdered form.

I need to be honest though. When I pulverized my kale it amazed me at how many large leaves fit into a small pint jar. The trouble was it smelled exactly like fish food. So, it still sits there. If you're not up for eating fish food (powdered kale), I won't tell. We'll let that be our little secret.

As to kale chips, wash the leaves and cut into 2" sections. Remove larger stems. After washing, spin them dry in a salad-spinner. To make chips, pour a light coating of olive oil over them and sprinkle with sea salt. Dry approximately four to five hours at 125 degrees. Now you're ready to eat healthy chips.

To dry kale, wash and spin-dry the leaves. Remove any tough stems if the plant has gotten large. If your leaves are too big to place into the dehydrator, slice them into two to three inch pieces. Dry at 110 degrees for approximately six hours. Store in an air-tight jar.

Spinach

Dried spinach makes a very useful powder. Added to pizza dough, homemade pasta, ricotta filling for lasagna or manicotti, homemade bread or as part of a sour cream (or sour cream/mayonnaise) dip, spinach offers a lot of options. Chopped and dried spinach can be a tasty addition to Italian sauces as well.

Wash the spinach and dry in a salad-spinner. It can be coarsely chopped or dried whole. Dry for six hours at 110 degrees.

All leafy vegetables and herbs can burn quickly. Watch them carefully and use lower settings on your dehydrator. There is a distinct difference between dried and burned and you'll know it when you see it. Be aware and check the drying progress periodically.

People in my classes frequently ask me if it is possible to burn items in the dehydrator. Yes, it is possible! And as you might expect, the more delicate the item or finely chopped, the more likely it is to burn if left too long. You'll know it once you see it too. The edges turn brown and if rehydrated, remain brown. Watch shredded foods and herbs especially closely.

Squash

This category has a lot going on. We can list many varieties of squash and all of them yummy. The idea is to consider what your favorites are and then how to dehydrate them. I mention pumpkin, butternut squash and zucchini but the possibilities are truly endless. They'll all be processed the same way: remove the skin before or after cooking, prepare the flesh, blanch (only if you removed the skin before cooking) and dry. Any squash that has a firm flesh will dehydrate well. Store in air-tight containers.

Pumpkin

I love pumpkin pie, and I'd always heard that pumpkin pie made from actual pie pumpkins (as opposed to canned pumpkin) is far superior. I love the idea of cooking from scratch but the thought of cooking a pumpkin from start to finish….bake it, cut it, scoop it, cook it, and finally eat it…each and every time seems a bit daunting. And if you know anything about me, I'm likely to start making pumpkin pie by planting the pumpkin seeds as well.

The perfect solution appears to be dehydration.

Purchase several pie pumpkins (or pull them out of your garden or compost pile…hey, it's been known to happen!) since the work is easier accomplished in mass. Bake the pumpkin in the oven or cook it in a pressure cooker. I enjoy using my pressure cooker since the food cooks quickly and without heating up the kitchen as much.

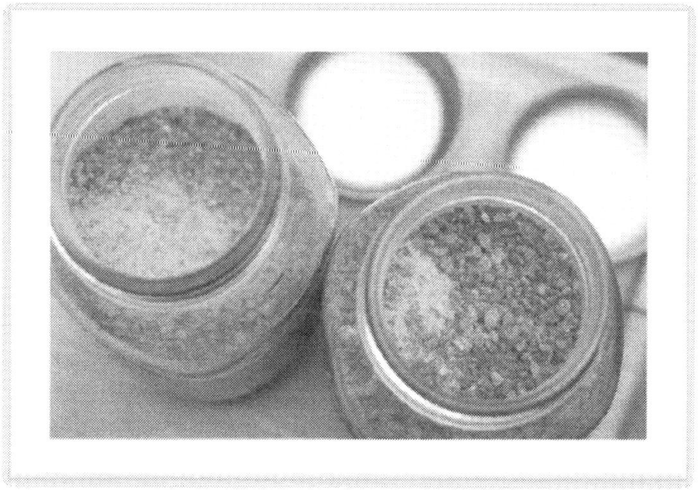

After cooking, slice open the pumpkin (which you'll find much easier now that it is cooked), remove the meat, separate out the seeds, and mash it to resemble mashed potatoes. Lay the pumpkin on parchment-covered racks. Gently press it down to a ¼" thickness. A lot of water will come out. If you choose not to use parchment paper or non-stick sheets, you'll have more trouble removing the pumpkin from the plastic racks. Consider yourself warned.

Dry the seeds on a separate rack and season lightly if desired.

As wet items like mashed pumpkin dries, it is probable that it will drip inside the dehydrator. Place a sheet of paper towel on the bottom for easier clean-up later. Dry the mashed pumpkin at 130 degrees for six to eight hours. At this point you can either store the pumpkin in large cracker size portions or you can pulverize it to powder for the easiest method of storing. I always store mine in powder form in my canning jars. One year I processed ten pie pumpkins and they all fit in one quart jar. You really have to see it to believe it.

If you have a favorite recipe that calls for canned pumpkin, try this instead. Mix ½ cup of pulverized pumpkin-powder with 2 cups of water when making a pie (use the standard pumpkin pie recipe with the substituted homemade puree) or for pumpkin puree used in pumpkin cake. You'll enjoy the taste of home-cooked pumpkins without the demanding process. At a moment's notice, you'll be able to savor the goodness of real food.

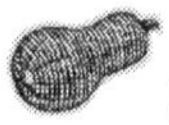

Butternut Squash

I've considered putting squash in the dessert section when I've worked on menu planning. Anything that creates a great pie like pumpkin or a yummy casserole like butternut squash should be treated with respect!

I generally process a bushel at a time. Using a potato peeler to remove the skin first I then chop it into squares since I like to store it best that way but I also prepare at least one quart jar worth of butternut powder, prepared exactly like the pumpkin.

After removing the skin, slice it or cube it and blanch for two to three minutes then submerge in cold water. If you cook it too long you'll be working with the mashed version which is perfectly acceptable, just different. Drain it well before placing it on the drying racks. Dry at 130 degrees for eight to ten hours.

When you're ready to use the squash, put ½ cup of the powder in a bowl and add two cups of boiling water. As it sits for twenty to twenty-five minutes, it reconstitutes itself into a lovely puree ready for baking or eating.

These powders are very useful in traditional dishes like pies, cakes, muffins and breads but are also quite handy in tasty autumn dips, soufflés, homemade baby food and healthy smoothies.

Zucchini

Zucchini is the vegetable that keeps on giving.

Your arms are loaded with zucchini from the garden, you're headed to a neighbor's house in the hopes of pawning off....ahem, I mean sharing your bounty, and you notice the window shades suddenly drop. Lights out. No one's home. Oh, really? So they don't want your leftover surplus either. Alrighty then. Head back to the kitchen, roll up your sleeves and get busy chopping and shredding. Zucchini is easy to dry, much easier than giving it away!

Zucchini can be dried with peel on or off, in slices or shredded. In powdered form it can be added to soups, stews, breads, rehydrated into baby food, added to meatloaf, or mixed into your next batch of homemade pasta….gourmet pasta anyone? Or it can be featured incognito in any dish feeding a picky eater who needs a boost of veggies in their diet. (Featured incognito? Is that even possible?) And that's just the powdered suggestions.

Sliced or shredded zucchini opens more doors of opportunity. Rehydrate the shredded for a great loaf of zucchini bread. Or make a batch of vegetarian lasagna and create a full layer of sliced or shredded zucchini. Add slices to soups or sauté as part of a medley of squash.

I prefer to dehydrate the smaller zucchini. If you're harvesting from the garden that means it is your job to check daily since zucchini grow from zero to sixty in one day….or something like that. We've all been surprised by the cave-man club of zucchini that just appeared overnight. Plan to shred the club should it make an appearance in your garden. Those tender little ones should be sliced. They end up looking like small dinner plates from a dollhouse. They're almost too cute to eat!

As with everything, slice zucchini evenly, place on trays, set the temperature at 130 degrees and the timer at seven to ten hours or two to three hours if you've shredded it. Since you'll have a lot of water draining from shredded zucchini, set it in a colander and let it drain for a little while before drying. Press down on the zucchini to help release the water. Your dehydrator will thank you.

Embrace your zucchini….kind of like you embraced it when you carried it half-way across the street, only with more love now.

Tomatoes

I intentionally plant an abundance of tomatoes each year. We love the flavor that fresh tomatoes add to our cooking. They're ear-marked for an easy canning project but not all will end up in my water-bath canner. Tomatoes are very easy to dehydrate and can be stored as slices or as powder. Naturally, the most space-saving option is powdered tomatoes.

Thus far, I have discussed using powdered foods as a sneaky way to include nutrient-dense foods in cooking. The soups and stews, though void of "unidentifiable chunks" still tout the health benefits we desire since the powder has enriched the dish.

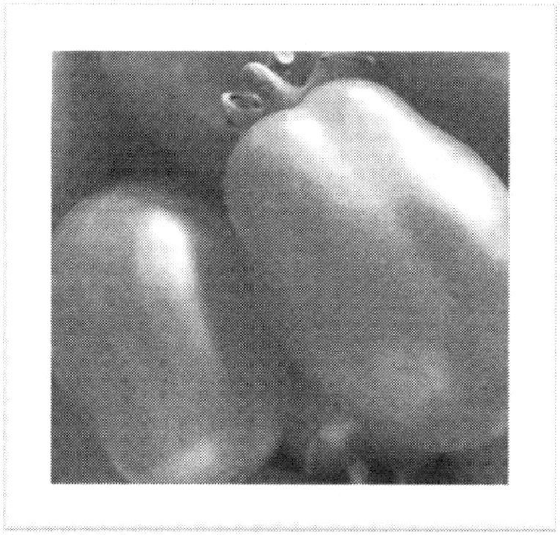

In the case of the acclaimed love apple, pulverized powder becomes extremely useful. Consider rehydrating the powder with less water for tomato paste. More water used will produce a tomato sauce and even more water, tomato juice. Add the home-grown herbs you've dried to the powder for a seasoned version. Put the powder in your cooking to thicken sauces and gravies or use in pasta and bread dough. The taste of tomato is delightful but nothing beats a tomato from your own garden. Imagine what the taste will do to your breads and pastas.

Tomatoes blend well with many things and your garden can be filled with a variety of them. Heirloom tomatoes come in a large assortment of colors and flavors. Now you have a way to preserve all of that taste, nutrition and goodness!

Tomatoes are high in lycopene so you'll want to add them to your diet frequently. If you dry them at 115 degrees or lower, you can use them in a veggie smoothie for enzyme benefits that can't be beat.

Plan to use the slices, whole or broken in stews, soups or sauces. Rehydrate and add to the top of pizzas or in casseroles. Thicken sauces with tomato powder.

To prepare, wash and core tomatoes. Slice ¼" thick and dehydrate for twenty to twenty-four hours at 130 degrees (or lower for a raw food). This may seem like a long time but foods with more water content require more time for complete drying. The juicier the tomatoes call for longer drying times and give less overall flavor than a meatier tomato. Roma tomatoes are my favorite variety to can and dehydrate. You'll know they're dry when they bend like leather and there is no moisture present.

When drying cherry or grape tomatoes, simply slice them in half and place the skin side down on the tray then dry at 130 degrees for twenty to twenty-four hours. These are a tasty garnish on salads.

If you use your tomatoes to make homemade ketchup, you'll want a great recipe to showcase the outstanding flavor. Years ago we started a tradition in our family of putting Love Sauce on our burgers. Now you can enjoy it too!

But first you need to know how to make homemade ketchup. When making ketchup, tomatoes are often cut, allowed to drain excess water, chopped, and cooked down. The mixture has to be pureed to achieve a smooth texture then the desired spices can be added and cooked till well blended.

Dehydrated tomatoes which have been pulverized mean you can start with a smooth texture and skip the tedious process of slicing, draining, chopping, and reducing. All you need do is add warmed water to the tomato powder and blend well in a pot while heating.

This is not a recipe. It is a suggested way of creating your own sauce. You'll decide how much to start with based on how much you use. And you may want a few small bowls around as you begin to experiment with the spices. Make a few concoctions to determine your personal favorite.

Begin with the tomato powder and warm water and slowly mix the two until you have the consistency and quantity you want. Start mixing slowly, knowing that you can always add more water or powder later. I start by pouring the powder into a bowl and then adding warm water gradually while stirring constantly.

The ketchup is now ready to be flavored. Once you've reached the texture and thickness you like, add the spices your family likes. Experiment. Common spices include: onions and bell peppers (use the dried, pulverized onions and peppers from your stash), garlic, salt, cayenne pepper, black pepper, paprika, ground cloves, celery seeds, mustard seeds, cinnamon, allspice, brown sugar, honey, and apple cider vinegar.

When adding spices, continue to cook slowly and stir constantly. The sauce will slightly thicken as it cooks. Store in the refrigerator.

Now it is time for me to tell you a story about Love Sauce.

Love Sauce

A story by Jan Nellis,

AKA "Love Means Never Having To Say You Have No Ketchup"

Once upon a time, in a very big city, there was a fast-food place where a young girl liked to eat. There were only two in this very big city and they were quite a distance from one another but both were very tasty and enjoyed by the girl.

Like a creature of habit, the girl always bought the same thing. A grilled burger on a lightly toasted bun with grated cheddar cheese and sauce. Oh, the Sauce. Happiness joined these two: the juicy burger and the yummy Sauce. And when the girl ate there, she joined in the happy union....and savored the moment.

Then one day the girl moved away.

Far, far away. Like when you discover it's hard to visit as often as you'd like and your heart starts hurting.

The body can always move. The heart often remains.

The girl decided that life was going to be only as good as she could make it so she set out to make it tasty.

Tasty is important. Never forget that.

Burgers, even juicy ones, can be made. Lightly toasted buns, grated sharp cheddar cheese....all these things can be had. But the Sauce!

So....on a dark and foggy night the girl set out to reunite herself with the moment of Happiness between Juicy Burger and Sauce.....as they had come to be known.

Call it fate. Call it destiny. Call it desperation on a mission. Yummy Sauce was achieved and forevermore became known far and wide as **LOVE SAUCE**! (Can you hear the angels singing???)

Love Sauce....a hush falls over the room.

Love Sauce...the mouth begins to water.

Love Sauce....a smile escapes the lips.

Love Sauce....Reunited with the Juicy Burger!

And now, many years later after a long bout of soul-searching, the girl, almost as young as she was in the former days.....only younger now because of the joy in her heart, decided to share this piece of Happiness with you.

You will accomplish this great feat with unexpected ease. You will pass it on to future generations. You will slather it on your burgers and pile high the mountain of grated cheddar cheese. You will become known far and wide for your great culinary skills. You will sing my praises...if you don't happen to already. And you will shout with exclamations of joy when the Great Burger Day comes and you can once again make Love Sauce.

Let us get down to business now. Are you prepared to begin impacting the world with more love?

Assemble your supplies and start your engines.

You'll need only a few things to make your great mark in the *Book of Tantalizing Tastes*:

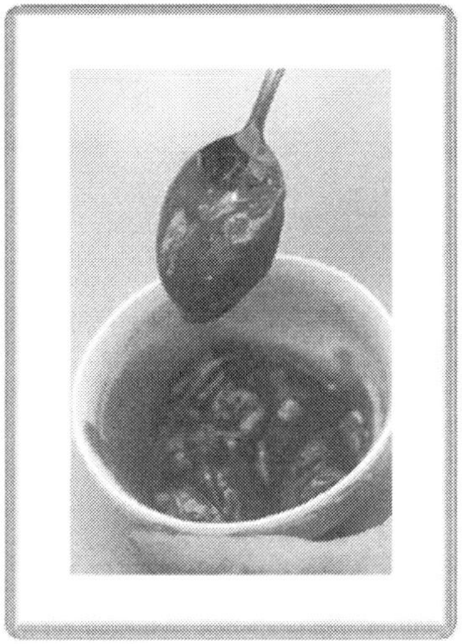

- 1 cup of ketchup
- 3 T. liquid smoke
- Bowl and spoon

Mix the two together until they are one. Lick spoon. You're done.

You are now a Graduate of my **Tantalizing Taste School for Masters**. What? Did you forget to send in the application for acceptance to this great school no-one-anywhere-has-ever-heard-about? Did you ***not*** enclose your check or money order? Are you suggesting you just got all this *for free*???

I guess I'll let you slide this *one time*....if you make a deal with me. Use my Great and Wonderful recipe frequently and herein and forevermore refer to it as the great Love Sauce that it is and spread your fair share of love in this world. The Good Lord knows we sure need it!

A message from the Dean of Culinary Education (that's me after all)**:** You may at any time adjust the measurements given. I just wanted to get you on a roll. More, less, whatever you want. You're the Boss; I only pretend to be the Boss. I found out I don't really like being the Boss. It's too demanding and *bossy*. It really doesn't pay that well either~

Mushrooms

I didn't always love mushrooms but I do now. I'm frequently buying fresh mushrooms, using what I can in salads, on pizza or on a crudités. Leftovers are quickly dried and sit in a jar on my cabinet. My children often throw a few into their ramen noodles (as well as peppers, onions or other dried options). The boiling water cooks them as it cooks the noodles. I'm also happy to rehydrate a few and throw them on a pizza when I have no fresh ones.

Mushrooms are the famous ingredient in many recipes. Think stroganoff, spaghetti sauce, rich gravies, Salisbury steak, chicken Marsala and you'll remember the role mushrooms play. But consider what a mushroom powder will do to add flavor to some of your favorite dishes. And when you'd like that mushroom presence without the visual (think: "Mom, you know I hate mushrooms!"), add the powder. Powdered mushroom equals my idea of the perfect compromise.

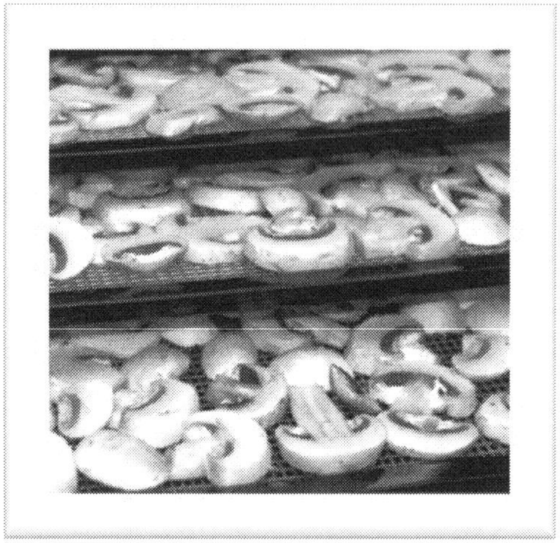

Now that you're wondering what else can possibly be said about mushrooms, wait, there's more! When I rehydrate mushrooms, the liquid left behind is a flavorful broth not to be wasted. Depending on what I'm cooking, I may choose to use it in the dish itself. In case you haven't noticed, I don't believe in wasting. "Waste not, want not" never goes out-of-date.

To prepare mushrooms for dehydration, gently clean and slice ¼" thick. Spread on drying racks and dehydrate at 130 degrees for eight to twelve hours. When mushrooms are dry they'll bend slightly with no moisture present. Store in an air-tight jar and have them handy for people who want to dress up something with extra flavor at the last minute.

Potatoes

Potatoes are great whether sliced, cubed or grated. I keep some of each on hand for use in various recipes. They rehydrate and cook perfectly. Plan to process them by peeling (removing any of the green flesh) then slice, chop or grate. Blanch first by adding to boiling water for five minutes. This will gently cook them. If you go longer than five minutes you will cause them to cook to mash and crumble. Remove with a slotted spoon and add to cold water. After cooling, dip potatoes briefly in a solution of ¼ lemon juice to ¾ water.

I prefer to process potatoes in large batches. Simply set up a work-station of sorts and work through the steps. You'll eventually have potatoes in all stages: some waiting to be peeled, a batch blanching, others soaking in the lemon/water solution, and sliced or cubed potatoes ready for trays. Since each step moves fairly fast, extra hands are an added asset. Here is your opportunity to convert a neighbor, friend or family member to the convenience of preserving food through dehydration.

My favorite recipe is scalloped potatoes. The potatoes are already sliced and waiting since I've dehydrated them fresh from the garden. I need only prepare my sauce and seasonings. This dish goes together easily and is enjoyed by all.

Scalloped Potatoes

- 3 cups dried, sliced potatoes rehydrated in 5 cups water
- ¼ cup dried, chopped onions rehydrated in ½ cup water
- 6 T. butter
- 6 T. all-purpose flour
- 1 t. salt
- Salt and pepper
- 3 cup milk
- 2 ½ cups cheddar cheese

Preheat oven to 400 degrees and butter a casserole dish. Layer half of the potatoes in the dish and add onions. Sprinkle with a layer of cheese. Top with remaining potato slices.

To make the sauce, melt the butter in a pan and mix in the flour stirring constantly with a whisk. Gradually add the milk. Continue to cook until the mixture has thickened. Stir in the cheese and continue stirring until fully melted. Pour the cheese sauce over the potatoes and cover the dish with foil. Bake for 1 ½ hours. Serves 5 - 6

Sweet Potatoes

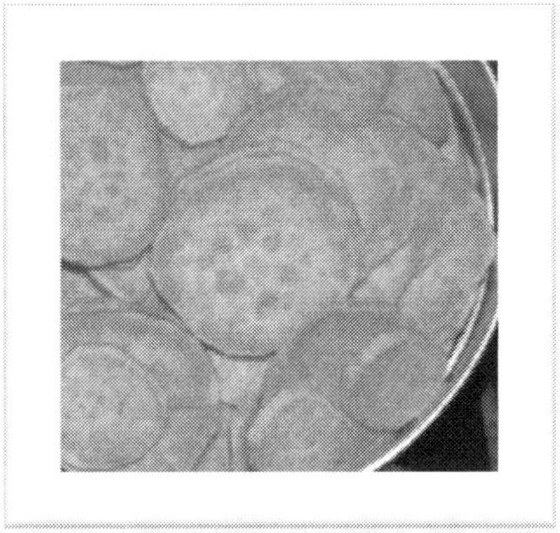

Sweet potatoes are processed exactly the same way as regular potatoes. All potato varieties dry beautifully. The meat of the potato becomes translucent and is considered dry when it is brittle and snaps when broken. And even though I've mentioned peeling the potatoes, it isn't necessary. I love potato slices with the peels still on them. The addition of the peel creates visual interest.

I have used the sweet potatoes to make traditional Thanksgiving casserole. I added pecans and dried cherries and they were wonderful. Try out some of your favorite dishes and see what you think.

I have sliced and cubed sweet potatoes. The cubed potatoes get rehydrated and mashed. And either sweet potatoes, yams or regular potatoes can be dried and crushed to powder. You've seen potato flakes....now you can make your own! Lastly, many people make sweet potato slices for dog treats. If you prefer to give your dog healthy fare, you now have the added option of making it yourself.

4 Fruit

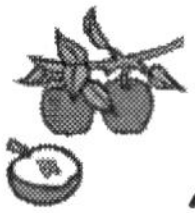

Apples

When autumn arrives and your favorite variety is ripe, buy a few pounds and prepare a healthy treat no one will refuse. I bought more than a bushel last year and I could have bought more. They are the perfect snack for road trips and are wonderful to cook with during the off-season.

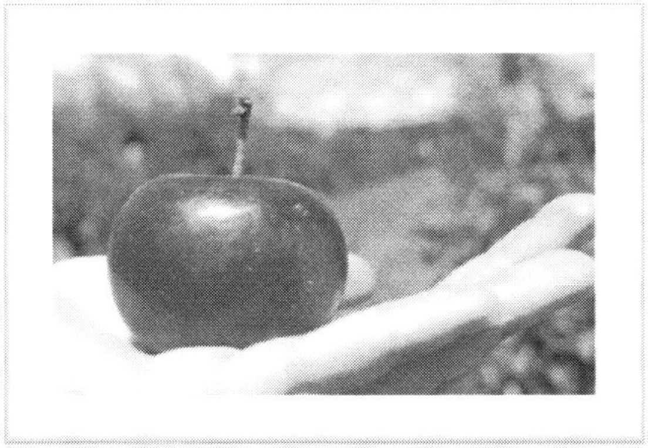

Apples can be dehydrated with the skin on or off... your

preference. Wash, core and slice the apples. When slicing any food for dehydration, all slices must be cut as uniformly as possible. Apples should be ¼" to ½" thick. Briefly soak the slices in a lemon bath. I suggest ½ cup of lemon juice to 6 cups of water. This prevents the natural browning that commonly occurs.

I save the peelings and dehydrate them as well. They'll go into my homemade tea bags as a base for apple cinnamon tea. After dehydrating the peeling, I put them in my blender and puree them. They're stored in a jar until I'm ready to put together the tea.

Place the apple slices on your trays without overlapping them. The small space between slices allows for air flow and even dehydrating. I like to lightly sprinkle them with cinnamon (no sugar!) though I generally do half with cinnamon and half without.

You can dehydrate apples at 130 to 135 degrees or as low as 115 degrees. The lower the temperature, the longer the drying period. Lower temperatures will require more time but gives a finished product that is still considered "raw food." As a family we are consciously making an effort to include more raw "living" foods in our diet for health benefits. Dehydration will allow you to preserve many foods still in their raw state.

The exact drying time will always vary based on how many trays you have prepared and how thickly you've cut your food item. Do not cut thin slices simply for the sake of a quick dry. Do so because you desire something more akin to a crispy cracker. Thicker apple slices are slightly chewy. Warning: While you are dehydrating apples, your house will smell like the House of Homemade Apple Pies, your friends and family will want a constant supply (think: Thanksgiving and Christmas homemade treats!) and you'll be tickled pink to see your loved ones eating a snack that is GOOD for them!

When rehydrating your apples, some water will remain after the apples have soaked up most of the liquid. It isn't just water anymore. It is now the makings of a lovely tea. Pour the water off by straining into a mug, add a touch of honey and relax while dinner is in the oven. It's like your own little reward built right into your cooking!

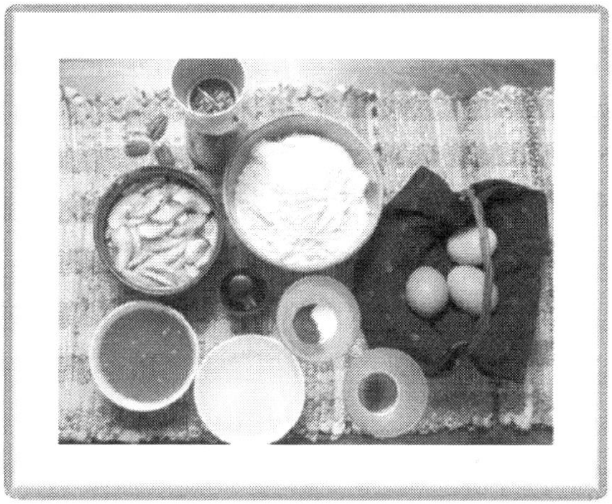

Try this tasty apple pancake with your dried apple slices:

German Apple Pancake

- 3 eggs
- ¾ cup milk
- ¾ cup flour
- 3 T. butter, divided
- ½ t. salt
- 1/3 cup honey
- 2 cups dehydrated apples rehydrated with 3 cups of water
- A sprinkle of nutmeg and cinnamon

Heat oven to 450 degrees.

Mix eggs, milk, flour, and salt. Stir in ½ cup of apples. Melt 2 tablespoons butter in a 12" cast iron skillet or oven-proof dish. After melting the butter and heating the pan, pour in the egg mixture and put into the oven for fifteen minutes. Turn the oven down to 350 degrees and continue to bake for ten minutes.

While the pancake bakes, melt 1 tablespoon butter in another pan and add the remaining apples and warm thoroughly. Sprinkle the apples with cinnamon and nutmeg. Remove the pancake from the oven and spread the warm apples gently over the pancake. Slice and serve.

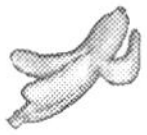

Bananas

I must admit I've never liked dried bananas from the grocery store. I wasn't planning to make any at home for that very reason. I thought I knew what dehydrated bananas tasted like so why bother. Thankfully the two are miles apart.

Add them to a trail mix or rehydrate them and mash them for banana nut bread or muffins. Use them in your pancake batter or cooked in steel-cut oatmeal.

On their own, bananas will turn an ugly brown. Slice and dip them in a lemon and water mixture. Place on a drying rack without overlapping and dehydrate at 130 degrees for six to ten hours or at 110 degrees for raw food. Bananas will bend slightly when dry and may be slightly sticky.

Berries

For such a small fruit, berries can be quite challenging. Blueberries are a delight to me but I'd rather make a fruit leather with them then go through the process of piercing each one to allow the moisture to evaporate.

In the case of any berry that is "sealed" you may find that even after hours and hours of dehydrating, they're still not dry. There's your cue to make leather. Whatever you decide, don't give up on berries.

Raspberries and blackberries are easier to dry. Just stand them up and dry at 130 degrees for twenty to twenty-four hours. Or enjoy health benefits with some great raw food and dehydrate them at 110 degrees for twenty-four to twenty-eight hours.

Strawberries

Strawberry season and I are close friends. We look forward to seeing one another. I say sweet things to the strawberries like: "You're so cute," or "I love you," or "How would you like to live in my backyard?" and the strawberries are flattered and act coy. They send up little white flowers and I can tell they want to talk to me too but just don't know what to say. I buy them…carton after carton, and we eat strawberry shortcake, strawberries and whipped cream, strawberry muffins and strawberries off our backyard plants. I've even made strawberry butter to put on pancakes. Oh, Baby.

Ultimately one of the best uses for dehydrating is the opportunity to dry foods you've grown yourself. Several years ago my husband built a strawberry pyramid. We grow our own strawberries and they send off runners so our harvest grows each year. You can build them to suit your purposes as long as each level gets slightly smaller as it goes up. Be sure to allow for enough plant room and then plan to dry your bounty!

Don't limit yourself. Put those yummy red bits into cake and muffin batters, rehydrate them (on a winter day!) and add them to angel food cake, surprise a little person with strawberry pancakes or put them in your new personalized tea bags.

I'd thought about sticking to fresh strawberries but dehydrated strawberries sounded like they'd be so good in trail mix. Watch out! They're tart! Slice them in ¼" pieces and dry them at 130 degrees for twelve to sixteen hours. Strawberries are a good candidate for raw snacks too. Adjust your temperature to 110 degrees and dry for fourteen to eighteen hours.

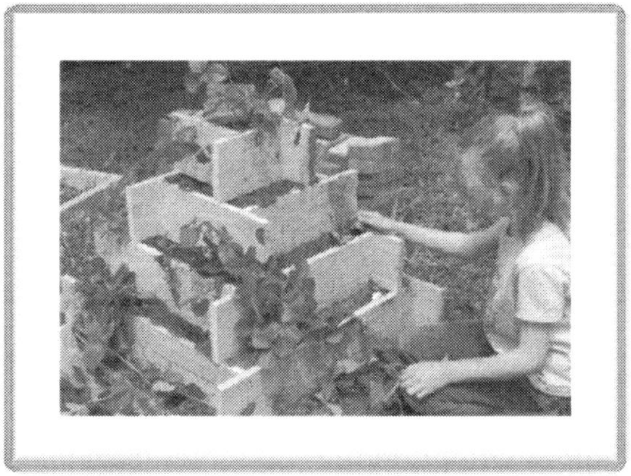

You'll love the chance to enjoy strawberries anytime of the year, especially if they've come out of your garden. If you haven't already, make friends with strawberry season this year.

Citrus

Lemons, limes, oranges, tangerines, satsumas, and grapefruit are all beautiful when dehydrated. The centers will darken but the flavor remains. I am particularly fond of some of the varieties that are harder to come by and now I enjoy them year-round.

I use dried citrus circles in glasses of water or in a large carafe for refreshing drinks without the calories. A decanter of color is inviting and thirst-quenching. Dehydrated citrus fruits are also lovely in garlands or wreaths during the holidays.

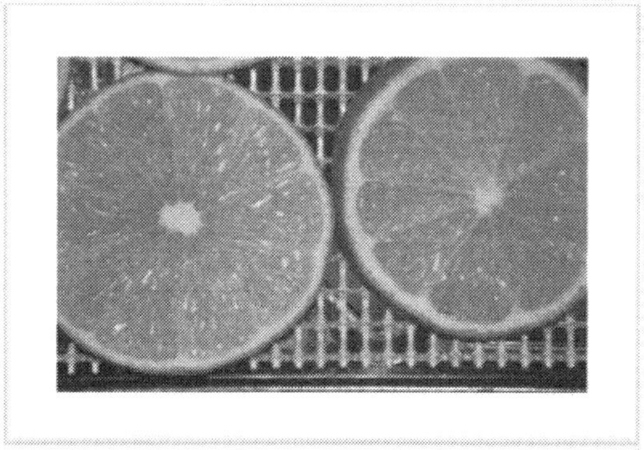

Citrus takes a little extra time when drying since they are primarily juice. You may even want to flip the slices on the tray to expose both cut sides to as much air as possible.

Wash the fruit before slicing since the peel will remain attached. Scrub it well and slice ¼" thick. Place on the trays without overlapping and dry at 130 degrees for approximately twenty-four hours. Test the slices by pinching the centers to feel for juice. If necessary, dry longer.

Cranberries

One year I took dried cranberries on a Thanksgiving family trip. The day was a potluck adventure and one of the items I was responsible for was the cranberry dressing. No canned sauce for me! (Forgive me if you love the jelled-in-a-can stuff!) Cooking up a delicious and traditional addition to the meal was nearly effortless and what fun I had in someone else's kitchen since I was prepared with dehydrated cranberries.

Don't attempt to dry whole cranberries. It won't be pretty. The berry is "sealed" and that seal needs to be broken first. I just know that some of you daredevils will be trying to dry whole berries. Go for it, Baby! Call me after you've cleaned things up. We'll talk.

You can painstakingly slice each berry in half, lay them on the trays skin side down (are you beginning to despair as you ponder the workload?) and dehydrate or you can break the seal the quick and easy way. Wash them, pop them in your blender, give them a quick spin and spread them out on the racks. I generally find a few that managed to get away (something like my father's old fishing days) so they get pulled out, run through the blender again and the drying process begins. I mentioned using them on Thanksgiving with the standard turkey meal but they're also perfect in a cranberry-orange nut bread or pulverized to use in homemade tea bags for cranberry tea (hot or cold).

Peaches

A part of me cringes when I dehydrate peaches. Much of the beauty of this sweet fruit is the juice that runs down your arm as you eat it. Yet drying it does have its rewards.

Peaches can be part of a trail mix or rehydrated and added to breads, muffins and cakes. Or you may decide to process them to a powder and stir into smoothies or baked items. Then again you could add them in powdered or sliced form to your own designer teabags for a hot or cold sensational drink. Peaches are a wonderful addition to homemade ice cream. You can add them rehydrated for bits of peaches or powdered for a more subtle, smooth flavor.

As with everything, slice peaches in uniform fashion, ¼" thick. Place on drying racks without overlapping and dry at 130 degrees for eight to twelve hours. The juicier they are, the longer they'll take to dry. If you plan to eat them in a trail mix, dehydrate for longer at 110 degrees to retain the healthy enzymes. Your body will thank you.

Pineapple

If you're looking for a sweet fruit to steal the show, you've found it. Pineapple takes everyone by surprise and I end up looking for a new hiding place. Well, it isn't really that bad. But almost. Yellow discs of happiness will tease your taste buds and keep you coming back for more. Slightly chewy, even the texture is appealing.

Raise the bar when you add dried pineapple to trail mix and don't forget the classic dessert: pineapple upside down cake. Finely chopped pineapple will add a hint of the tropics to your tea bags and when making fruit leathers, mix ¼ cup of ground, finely chopped pineapple with the main fruit to help preserve the naturally bright color.

Before we talk about how to cut and dehydrate a pineapple, you should be made aware of the fact that you'll actually need two pineapples for the full experience. Let's be honest. You're going to eat half of everything you cut. They're irresistible. So go ahead and get two. You'll have one to dry and use later and one to eat and share now. (That sharing part is purely optional.)

If you want to make your mark in the world by becoming a Dehydrated-Pineapple Specialist, buy a pineapple slicer. It will slice the fruit, remove the core and put you on the top-ten list of world famous pineapple-slicers. If your phone starts ringing nonstop, don't blame me.

I like to cut my pineapple so I have complete rings to dehydrate. But you can cut it up lengthwise to end up with chunks. Either works well. Start with a ripe pineapple and slice the top off. Cut the pineapple into ¼" slices or cubes by carefully removing the outer skin and cutting away the inner core. Place the pieces on a rack and dry at 130 degrees for twelve to sixteen hours. (For raw dried pineapple, dry no hotter than 110 degrees and add a couple of hours to the wait.) Pineapple will be leathery when completely dried. Store in an air-tight container....and hide it!

Fruit Leather

Making fruit leather is easy and much less expensive than purchasing the store version. If you're interested in having something without preservatives in the fruit of your choice, make some in your dehydrator.

We're fortunate enough to have property where fruit trees can be grown. If you have fresh fruit just waiting to be used, set some aside for drying and put some in the blender for leather.

Personally, I don't like to add too much additional sweetener. I feel like the fruits tend to be so sweet themselves (especially when completely ripe) that I hate to take away from their goodness by adding sugar. In fact, I don't add sugar at all. I try to limit the amount of sugar we eat under normal circumstances and since we happen to be beekeepers, we opt for honey.

Use ripe fruit, cut away any blemishes and pulverize them in a food processor. Adding a little crushed pineapple will help them retain their beautiful color. If you'd like a touch of sweetness, add a tablespoon or so of honey. Don't add too much since it might prevent the fruit from completely drying. (Thank the bees while you're at it. They work awfully hard to get that for you.)

Dress up your leather with some spices like cinnamon with apples or a dash of lemon juice with blueberries or some homemade vanilla with bananas or peaches. If you pulverize nuts very finely, you can add them to the fruit as well. Stir a little shredded coconut into the puree.

Spread the fruit puree out on a non-stick sheet ¼" thick. Dry for eight to ten hours at 110 degrees for raw leather (that sounds exciting) or six to eight hours at 130 degrees. It is dry when there are no visible moist spots. Remove it while it is warm since it hardens slightly as it cools. Roll it up jelly-roll style in plastic wrap or parchment paper so it doesn't stick to itself. Store it in an air-tight container at room temperature.

Think about making some exotic flavors like a tropical mix of mangoes, pineapples, bananas and strawberries. Or put some peaches and cherries together for a delightful taste-combination. Strawberries and bananas are famous friends and they make delicious, chewy leather.

When deciding how much of this or that to use, be very flexible. Use the fruit you have and blend it well, add a very small amount of liquid if it doesn't have much natural juice (it isn't necessary but may come in the form of honey, lemon, orange or pineapple juice) and spread it out until you've got it all on trays.

This isn't a recipe to hold you back and force you to use exact quantities. It is meant to give you freedom in your own kitchen. If you have a handful of ripe peaches, make leather. If you have a basket of sweet strawberries or a blueberry bush bursting with berries, make leather. Fill the trays till you run out of puree and enjoy the fruits of your labor.

Homemade Gold Label Vanilla

I know. I just read your mind. You want to make homemade vanilla now, don't you?

Vanilla extract is easily purchased from the grocery store. So why make it yourself? Because you can. And because it's fun.

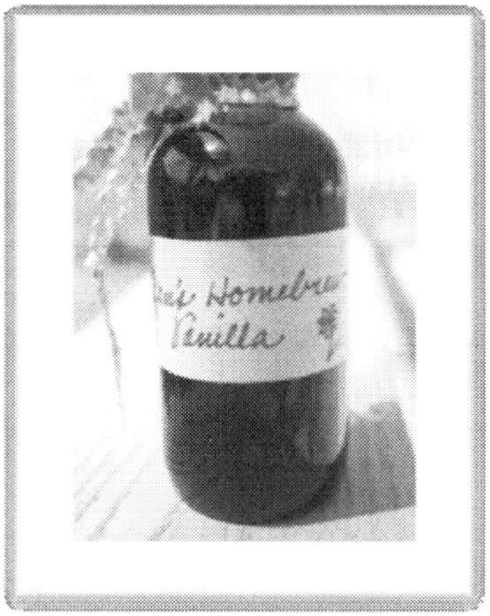

You'll want the vanilla tincture to sit for the full six weeks but I like letting mine sit for up to six months. You call that stuff: Gold Label Vanilla.

You'll need some top-quality vanilla beans. (I get mine online.) I also prefer to buy organic. You can pick from a variety of beans. Decide what you'd like or purchase a variety. You'll need six beans per cup of vanilla and I always make large batches since I like having some on hand to give away. The little amber bottles make perfect gifts to put in a basket of cooking supplies.

Begin by pouring rum or vodka into a large quart or half gallon canning jar. I use the best rum I can buy. Remember: good ingredients make good food. You're going to make this batch in a large jar and then pour it off into smaller jars once it has cured.

For every one cup of alcohol you poured, add six vanilla beans that you have cut open. I slit the bean lengthwise, scrape out some of the seeds with a spoon and add the seeds and beans to the alcohol. Screw on the lid and shake with wild abandon. Store the bottle in a cabinet where it can sit for at least six weeks. Shake the jar once a day. I always put a little note on the inside of the cabinet door so I'll remember what day I made it and what day it is fully cured.

When you're ready to use this delightful vanilla, buy some small glass amber bottles and using a funnel, pour the vanilla until it is approximately ¾ full. Next, add a couple of vanilla beans (you may need to slice them into shorter sections since the bottles are small) and top it off with more vanilla. Seal and label so your friends will know what they're getting. Keep a stash for yourself. You're ready to start the next batch now. By starting now, that six-month wait won't seem so bad.

When I was a little girl, as my mother and I were baking, we always wished there was a vanilla perfume. I know it seems unheard of now to wish for such a thing when vanilla items abound. From candles to perfume, from soaps to air-fresheners, vanilla fragrance is an option in just about anything. And almost everyone likes it. I smile to myself as I make homemade vanilla now. We add it to all of our baking, some of our smoothies and leathers, tea bags for hot or cold tea, homemade ice cream and a splash to a pot of steel-cut oatmeal. Talk about good. It's an ingredient that I've become known for….

Have you ever had anyone tell you to buy the "good vanilla?" The point is, they want you to stay away from the chemically created vanilla. It may be cheap but it isn't vanilla. By using alcohol, you're creating a tincture and the rum or vodka pulls the essential oils from the beans and seeds giving you the essence of vanilla in liquid form. Obviously this is meant for cooking, not drinking.

Designer Tea Bags

You've learned how to dehydrate a wide variety of fruits now so you're ready to design some tasty tea bags. They are very easy to fill and you'll be renowned as the Master of Flavor. Empty tea bags can be purchased and sealed with an iron. Surprise someone with a taste for something wonderful to your custom tea bags.

If you make individual tea bags, use a total of one to one and a half teaspoons of leaves and flavorings. You can also make larger tea blends to use with a tea ball strainer. Store them in beautiful jars. Add a twist of lemon to the tea, a drop of cream or a touch of honey. You'll love the variety you can create.

Make each bag by mixing half tea leaves and half spice, fruit or both. Remember to include several varieties of teas as you create your blends. Pick from good quality black, green or white leaves or use the mint and raspberry leaves from the garden. Plan to mix in the zest of lemons, oranges, tangelos, clementines or satsumas. Pick fruit choices based on your favorites. Consider what you've already learned how to dry and what you like best. Choose from apples, pineapple, melons, kiwi, mangoes and peaches, or any berry such as blueberries, raspberries, or strawberries. Add small chopped up bits of high-end vanilla beans or a pinch of cinnamon or both if it sounds good! Hopefully you're getting the idea that this should be fun and creative. If you happen to make a blend you don't like, don't make it again. If you use all of your lemon zest, make some more!

Apples are a particular favorite of mine. I save the peel and dehydrate them. They go into homemade tea bags as a base for apple cinnamon tea. After the peel has been dried, I pulverize them. Mix apple peel with a dash of cinnamon and black or green tea leaves. The powder can be stored indefinitely in a jar until you're ready to put together the tea.

Raspberries can be dried along with the leaves for a delicious tea. Dry the leaves as you would any delicate herb.

Mint leaves which grow like wild-fire in gardens can be gathered and used for a simple tea. Keep the leaves as whole as possible while you store them so they crumble and release their flavor as the tea is made.

The peel of oranges and lemons when dried is pulverized and blended with black tea leaves to make invigorating beverages.

Ginger is ideal for settling a stomach and you can make that one from the gingerroot you've dehydrated for your herb collection. Mix the dried powder with black tea leaves and add a bit of lemon zest or fresh lemon juice.

You've always had tea as a beverage option. Now you can spice it up with something you've created yourself.

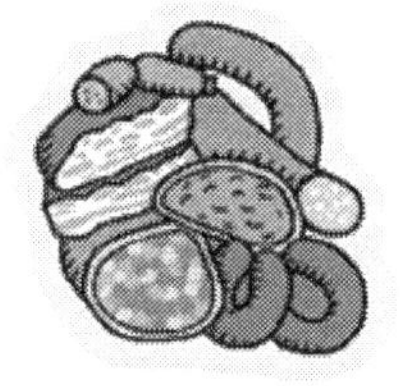

5 Jerky

One of the ultimate dehydrating experiences is preserving meat. It isn't difficult but you must follow certain rules to assure you've dried a wholesome product that will be safe for consumption.

The first thing to consider is that all meats used must be lean cuts. Before you begin the drying process, you must remove as much fat as possible. Fatty meat will spoil quickly and you want a meat that will last. There are several good choices to pick from:

- Eye of round
- Flank steak
- Lean ground beef
- Sirloin tip

Hunters often come home with a hefty supply of meat and not all of it need be frozen. Use the pieces suitable for dehydrating to make jerky. (You may also decide to can some of the meat! Canning meat must be done in a pressure canner! Try not to count on your freezer….or the electric company….for all of your food preservation.)

Even after cutting the fat from your meat, you'll find that it will continue to "melt" out as you dry it. If this happens just blot it with a paper towel once it has finished drying.

The other aspect of drying meat has to do with whether or not you decide to precook the meat. You can cook the meat for a few minutes after removing it from the marinade and before placing it into the dehydrator or you can take it from the marinade and put it straight into the dehydrator. The meat will be dried at 155 degrees for many hours. It is actually being slow-cooked and dried at the same time. For the record, we don't pre-cook our meats although we aren't against the idea.

Another great aspect of drying meat is the variety of marinades you can use. You can purchase bottled marinades or envelopes of dry mixes you put together yourself. You'll find just about anything your heart desires. Of course my preferred method is making the marinade yourself.

If possible, partially freeze the meat before slicing it by placing it in a freezer for an hour or two. You'll find your meat is easier to work with if you cut it when it is almost solid. The strips of meat can be thinner as well. Cut the meat ¼" thick with the grain. Place in a quart-size zip-lock bag and pour the marinade over it. Let the meat sit in the marinade eight to twenty-four hours.

After soaking, pour the meat and marinade into a colander and drain. Place the meat strips on the drying racks and dry at 155 degrees for six to eight hours. The meat is dry when it is leathery. For brittle jerky, let it dry an additional two hours. Store in air-tight jars or in freezer bags. Jerky can be made in larger quantities and stored in the freezer in bags.

One additional option when making jerky involves applying Morton's preserving salt to the meat before placing it into the marinade. Rub the salt over the meat and let it sit for one hour per quarter-inch of thickness. After sitting, rinse the salt and place into the marinade and proceed as directed above.

Marinades aren't difficult to make. Whatever you consider good is what you should try to create. If you like spicy jerky, add dried cayenne peppers or pepper flakes. If you want a sweet flavor like teriyaki, add a little brown sugar, teriyaki sauce and some soy sauce. I enjoy the taste smoke sauce adds to meat. Cracked pepper and sea salt is a good and simple option. Fresh garlic powder, dried sage, chopped onions, dried oregano, parsley, dried or prepared mustard, apple-cider vinegar, lemon or pineapple juice, or honey are all possible additions. Use some of these ingredients to mix up custom batches of the jerky you'll soon become famous for. I simply want you to know that the ideas and possibilities are endless.

The amount of marinade you make will depend on the amount of meat you are drying. We tend to dry in batches of three pounds. Remember three to four pounds of meat will equal one pound of dried meat. But don't go crazy making jerky. Try a few recipes and decide what you enjoy before making larger batches.

I mentioned earlier that you can dry ground meat as long as it is lean. The marinade you prepare for your meat is thoroughly mixed into the ground meat which causes it to have a little more "staying power." Mix and let it sit for a little while then put it on the trays in strips you make yourself. This is where the jerky gun comes in handy. If you don't have one, do your best to create little strips similar to what you would make if you were cutting a piece of meat keeping it at ¼" thick. When ground beef becomes jerky it tends to crumble more when over-dried. I personally enjoy it since the flavor runs completely through the meat. Jerky made from ground meat is a bit more fragile. Keep this in mind when deciding which cut of meat you plan to use, how you intend to use it or store it.

Dried meat is generally eaten as jerky but if you're storing food for "a rainy day," consider using dehydrated meat in stews or soups. Meat can be rehydrated for cooking purposes and serves well as an additional item in your food pantry. I suggest eating it in a pot of something warm and soothing.

Grub Rub

- 3 pounds of lean meat sliced ¼" thick
- 2 t. sea salt
- 1 t. freshly ground black pepper
- ½ t. cayenne pepper

Combine the spices and rub on meat. Place in a zip lock bag and refrigerate for eight hours or overnight. Lay pieces on dehydrating racks and dry at 155 degrees for six to eight hours.

Aloha Jerky

- 3 pounds of lean meat sliced ¼" thick
- 1 c. finely chopped fresh onion or ½ c. dried onion rehydrated in 1c. boiling water
- ½ c. shredded pineapple
- 15 cloves garlic
- 3 T. honey
- 3 t. ground dried ginger
- 2 t. black pepper
- 1 t. sea salt
- ½ c. soy sauce
- ¼ c. apple-cider vinegar

Slice meat ¼" thick while partially frozen. Mix all marinade ingredients and place meat and marinade in zip-lock bag. Let it sit for eight hours or as long as overnight in the refrigerator. Place on the drying racks without touching and dry at 155 degrees for six to eight hours. Store in an air-tight container or in the freezer for longer storage.

Teriyaki Jerky

- 3 pounds lean meat
- 3 T. cornstarch
- 3 T. cold water

- ¾ c. honey
- ¾ c. apple cider vinegar
- 3 cloves garlic minced
- 1 ½ t. ground ginger
- 1 t. black pepper

Slice partially frozen meat into ¼" thick slices.

In a saucepan, combine the honey, soy sauce, vinegar, ginger, and black pepper. Bring to a boil over medium-high heat. While the sauce is heating, combine the cornstarch and cold water. Mix well with a fork or whisk. When the sauce comes to a full boil, add the cornstarch mix and stir until thickened and bubbly. Remove from the heat and let cool.

Once the teriyaki sauce has cooled, add the sliced meat and allow it to sit in the marinade eight hours or overnight in the refrigerator. Drain the meat and marinade mixture in a colander and place meat strips on a drying rack. Dehydrate for six to eight hours at 155 degrees. Store in an air-tight container or in the freezer for longer storage time.

6 Yogurt

Everything coming out of the dehydrator has been dry so far. Mission accomplished. But this time we're talking about how to use the dehydrator for something else entirely.

We're not looking at this appliance as something to remove moisture. We're considering it as a way to maintain a constant

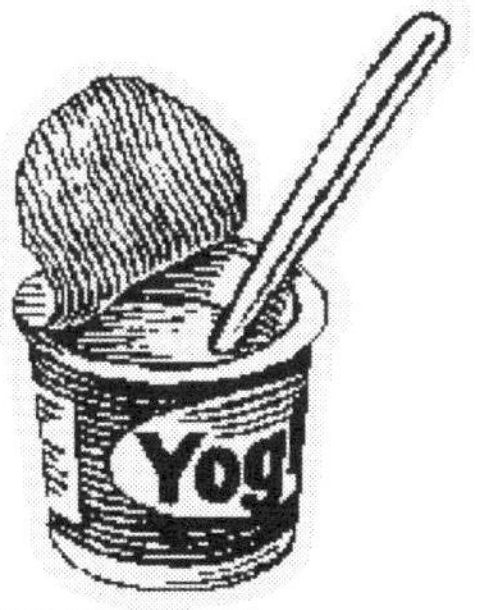

temperature. You may have thought about purchasing a yogurt maker in the past…or maybe you bought one. If you'd like to use your dehydrator to make yogurt, you'll need to use it without the trays. In this case, trays serve no purpose. You want the dehydrator, space to put the jars, and a steady temperature.

You can make yogurt with all types of milk. I use whole fat milk. I'm of the opinion that we need to be eating healthy fats. If you want to use low-fat milk, by all means do so. You'll also want a starter. Buy good yogurt. Look for something with active cultures in it. Get plain yogurt. You'll dress up the taste with flavors later.

You can purchase dry starter from health food stores or online. There are a lot of different choices. Yogurt has been around for many years! You can imagine the depth of information and resources available.

One of the most common starters is a Belgian starter. Its consistency closely resembles the yogurt you're used to, remains active so you can use it again as a starter and has a traditional taste. But don't hesitate to try something new.

Begin by assembling your equipment and ingredients:

- Quart or pint glass canning jars with lids
- Plain yogurt with active cultures
- Milk (whole or low-fat cow's milk or goat's milk)
- Powdered milk (optional)

- Large pot
- Thermometer

You'll want to begin by thoroughly washing your jars. Since you want good bacteria to grow you must be certain that clean conditions exist.

I prefer to measure out my ingredients based on how many jars I'm making. The idea here is that I measure the ingredients to fit the jars. I'm always confident that I know exactly how much yogurt I'm getting and am prepared with the proper number of washed jars.

How many jars are you making? Pour enough milk into your pot to fill the jars. Turn the heat to low and begin warming the milk. Now add one healthy teaspoon of your starter yogurt to each canning jar. You've just put the bacteria into the jar and you're about to give it a food source.

Some people add powdered milk to the liquid milk at this point. I've done so with good results. The purpose of the powdered milk is to make a smooth yogurt. Adding it is completely optional. If you do so, just whisk well to assure it has mixed thoroughly.

Meanwhile, heat the milk to the point of simmering. You may read that some people boil their milk. Milk is so unstable once it reaches the boiling point that you could end up with a nasty mess if you're not careful. I watch the pot and stop heating it just as it begins to reach the point of boiling. Turn off the heat and let the milk cool to between 115 and 118 degrees.

When you mix the warmed milk and your active bacteria, you'll want to be gentle. The bacteria are living and hot milk will kill them. Be certain that the milk has cooled to the proper temperature before mixing. Pour the milk into the jars and stir. I use a fork since it works like a mini-whisk. Screw the lids on and place in your dehydrator.

Set the temperature on the dehydrator to between 105 and 110 degrees. That setting will be warm enough for the proper growth to occur but not so hot as to kill it. Process the yogurt for six to eight hours. As tempted as you may be (I know I always am) don't disturb the jars!

Remove your yogurt after processing and look at the wonder and mystery that just occurred in your dehydrator. Milky goodness becomes thick and rich, good-for-you bacteria! What's not to like about that? Sound tasty?

Do you want flavor? Longing for something more than plain? Add your favorite fruits after you've completed the "dehydration process." Mix in anything from the jam you've canned yourself to maple syrup from a friend's harvest. Stir in chunky applesauce or a few spoons of Jan's Delicious Granola. Another tasty choice is a few drops of homemade vanilla. Our family favorite addition is honey from the bees we know and love.

It doesn't take much to dress up plain yogurt. You're not trying to cover the taste; you're trying to enhance it based on the mood you're in or the way you intend to use it.

Store the jars in the fridge and use a teaspoon of that yogurt to start your next batch. You can easily reuse this seed for five or six batches. It becomes apparent when the starter is weak and ready to be replaced.

If you've been preserving foods, chances are good you've come across raw milk. Maybe that's what you drink. We do. Raw milk is special. Never heated and containing lovely enzymes, it has a delightful taste and is creamy beyond compare. (Be aware that raw milk has not been pasteurized or homogenized. Cream will rise to the top and can be used to make butter. If you want pasteurized milk, raw milk is not for you!)

The key here though is that it has not been heated and you just read instructions that call for heating the milk. If you have plenty of raw milk from your family cow, feel free to heat it and make your yogurt. Bessie's got more where that came from! If you buy raw milk at a premium you don't want to heat the milk and sacrifice the very thing that sets it apart from other milk. First and foremost, be keenly aware of the sanitary conditions of your milk supplier. You don't want milk from anyone who has less than pristine standards….for drinking or cooking!

In an effort to preserve as many of the good qualities of raw milk, heat to 118 degrees and take it off the heat. Proceed with the instructions as described for standard yogurt. Powdered milk can be used in this recipe as well but I want my raw milk to be only raw milk. If you find it not as thick as you'd like, put the yogurt in a cheesecloth bag and drain some of the liquid off. Don't throw away the liquid. Your pets will love it and it is very good for them; or, use it in your cooking. Nothing about raw milk should be wasted!

How to drain the yogurt from a bag:

Put a piece of butter muslin or cheesecloth in a colander. Spoon the yogurt into the bowl. Grab the four corners of the fabric, lift and hang from a clothes hanger. Let it drain. The idea isn't to remove all of the liquid, just some of it.

We eat our yogurt with a wide variety of delicious goodies swirled in but we also use it in smoothies. Talk about good! Use plain yogurt in recipes that call for sour cream or mayonnaise. I'm not suggesting you spread it on a ham and swiss cheese sandwich but I do think you'll be pleased with the results if you replace a portion of the mayo with plain yogurt. Now you have one more healthy option up your sleeve.

Jonny Rex and the Fruit Smoothies

- 1 pint homemade yogurt
- Frozen strawberries
- Frozen bananas
- Frozen pineapple chunks
- 1 pint orange-pineapple juice

Put yogurt and juice in blender. Add generous portions of fruit. Blend until you've reached a smooth consistency. Add a tablespoon of coconut oil if desired. You'll have enough to enjoy and share!

Each time you make a smoothie, you'll have a different creation. You want something cold and tasty? Pull out your blender and whatever frozen fruit you currently have on hand. Throw in a little of this and a little of that. Smile as you hum a nice tune while moving across the kitchen floor. Something yummy is coming and you're making it yourself. As nice as those fancy fruit bars are, extra cash in your pocket is pretty darn nice too.

Additional fruits: blueberries, mangoes, peaches, raspberries or blackberries.

Jan's Delicious Granola

- Coconut oil to lightly coat pan
- 6 cups old fashioned oats
- ½ cup roughly chopped pecans
- ½ cup roughly chopped walnuts
- ½ cup sliced almonds
- ¾ cup honey
- ¼ cup molasses
- 2 T. homemade vanilla (or pure vanilla)
- 1 t. cinnamon
- ½ t. sea salt
- ½ c. coconut oil

Rub a thin layer of coconut oil on your baking sheet. Preheat the oven to 300 degrees. Mix the oats, nuts, salt and cinnamon in a large bowl. In a small pot, warm the honey, molasses and coconut oil. Simmer for five minutes. Remove from the heat and add the deliciously aromatic vanilla. Pour the sweet mixture over the oats while stirring. Finish blending by mixing with your hands if necessary. Spread granola on the baking sheet and bake for twenty to thirty minutes until golden brown. Let it cool completely before storing in an air-tight container.

My family just loves yogurt with granola. Yours will, too!

7 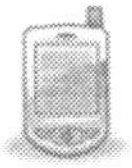 Miscellaneous Dehydrating Fun. Really.

I've dehydrated an odd assortment of things but late one evening I was given my most unusual and expensive item yet. Mess up a batch of carrots and you're out three bucks. Mess up on a four-hundred dollar iPhone and you're facing a lifetime of remorse and regret. You think that's a little high on the exaggeration-factor? Think again. Ask the teen or the parent that just bought the phone and you'll see what I mean. I'm tempted to call this section:

Everything You Always Wanted to Know about Dehydrating Your Phone but Were Afraid to Ask

Or,

How Your Dehydrator Can Pay for Itself in Just One Day!

What worked for us: Turn off the phone and put it into a large bowl of rice. Remove as many trays as necessary and put the bowl into the dehydrator. Set the temperature control to 140 degrees, set the timer to eight hours and pray. When it is dry it won't be crispy, it won't be leathery, and you need not store it in an air-tight container….but then again, given the fact that you just dropped it in water, maybe you should. And I'm saying that as sweetly as possible.

Hey folks, accidents happen. You may as well be prepared! I'm happy to report that the phone was in perfect working order following dehydration and it didn't just get wet, it got submerged! Wish I could make promises about events like this in the future. I just can't. What I can tell you is that it is worth a try.

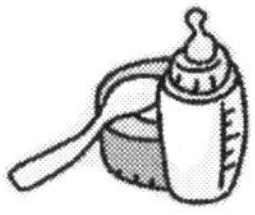

Baby Foods

As I mentioned earlier, I'm starting to go a little crazy about all of the modified foods. Dare I even call genetically modified items food? Now that we know the origin of Frankenfoods, is it mandatory that we eat them?

I know how hard it is to say no to something that is difficult to identify. If it isn't labeled how will you know when to pass it up? So instead of deciding what you won't eat or feed your baby, what if you focused on what you will eat or feed your baby?

Babies are such precious creatures and we want to give them the best as they begin growing. You can make your own baby foods buy purchasing or growing the foods you trust. Dehydrate the fruits and veggies that are age-appropriate for your child and then pulverize them into a powder. When you're ready to feed Little Baby, just rehydrate by adding hot water, letting it sit for fifteen to twenty minutes and then giving Junior a taste of the Good Stuff. (Always test the temperature of the food before feeding it to Baby. You don't want to burn a little mouth!)

I remember when my first child was a baby. I wanted to give him something to eat that he could get excited about. I made our beef stew from scratch and when he was able to eat each of the ingredients, I'd put his portion in my blender and create the famous baby-food texture. I froze his dinner size meal in the old Tupperware hamburger-patty containers. He'd eat each and every bite....licked the platter clean, so to speak. And I knew he was getting a sound diet of good foods.

Now as I look at the variety of foods which I dehydrate, I am constantly reminded of what great homemade and good-for-you baby food can be made in the dehydrator. I don't question whether or not the foods have been poisoned with spray-on treatments. I know the food that I have just prepared hasn't been preserved through radiation. What I've grown in my own garden or purchased from a reputable farmer's market is clean and ready to savor!

I want my children to be healthy and able to enjoy life. I need to feed them so they are prepared to do so. "Come, Baby, it is time to eat something good."

Nuts

If you'd like a healthy snack, consider nuts. They are extremely nutritious and full of flavor. Pecans, a prized-nut from the south, contain calcium, iron, magnesium, phosphorus, potassium, and selenium while cashews are rich in magnesium, phosphorus, and potassium. Macadamia nuts are a deliciously rich treat filled with iron, magnesium, phosphorus, potassium, zinc, and vitamin B.

Nuts contain phytic acid and enzyme inhibitors which make digesting them difficult. When phytic acid combines with the naturally occurring minerals in nuts, it interferes with the absorption process. You'll miss out on many health benefits.

In order to make the nutrients more accessible and the digestion process easier, soak the nuts in salt-water overnight first. After soaking, the nuts need only be dried in an oven or dehydrator until crispy and then they are ready to be enjoyed.

How to soak and dehydrate nuts:

Mix 4 cups of nuts with one tablespoon of salt and a quart of water. (You can also use whey or lemon juice in place of the salt.) Let them soak overnight and drain in a colander. Spread on the drying trays and dehydrate for twelve to twenty-four hours at 150 degrees. The nuts will be crispy when they are completely dehydrated. Store in an air-tight container.

Waldorf Salad

6 apples, chopped (I always use a mix of tart and sweet, red and green)

1 ½ c. chopped celery

¾ c. chopped crispy pecans or walnuts

½ c. sour cream

½ c. mayonnaise

1 ½ T. lemon juice

1 T. honey

Make the dressing by mixing together the sour cream, mayonnaise, lemon juice, and honey. Stir the apples, celery, and nuts into the dressing and chill for several hours before serving. Serves 6.

Vacation Alert

When we're planning to go out of town, I start going through the fridge. Normal protocol says you eat your perishables so you don't come home to a science experiment gone bad. But what if you can't eat it all? Does that mean it will be destined for the trash or compost pile? Naturally, the answer is no. Begin a week before your departure and start dehydrating the surplus.

I remember the day this plan occurred to me. I was so pleased that I'd found a solution which preserved my food. Throwing away food causes me great pain. You work for the money to buy the food, you pick it out, push it through the entire store, pay for it, load it into the car, unload it and store it and eventually cook it! After all that work you can't possibly throw it away. Be responsible with your resources: finances, time, food, or money. They're all extremely valuable.

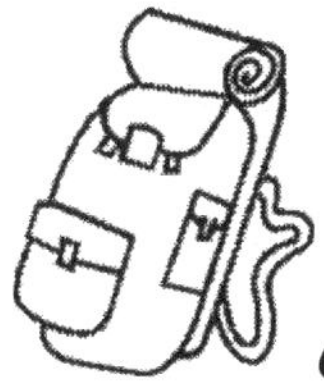

Camping

The first time I saw dehydrated foods was in little bags with big prices at a specialty store. Each package made a "delicious hot meal for the hungry hiker." I remember thinking it was a genius-idea....except for the expense and required purchase: one package for each person for every meal. Lightweight and portable, easy to prepare with few additional ingredients required, camping and hiking had a new appeal. I still see the beauty in such a plan but now I'm able to prepare those little pouch-dinners myself. I can even seal it with a simple food sealer in my own kitchen. A meal still light-weight and portable, still delicious, but now made with my ingredients and much more affordable.

Our family camps on a regular basis and it gives me the perfect chance to work on meal ideas to please a wide variety of tastes. I've even played with the notion of making a "Bike and Hike" meal for my son and his girlfriend with the instructions, "You hike and take great pictures, enjoy the beauty around you and be surprised and pleased with the gourmet fare to be enjoyed al fresco."

What about making your own camping or hiking meals? What if you could put together a nice dehydrated dinner for someone who loves the backwoods and forests? Stay clear of the pricy outdoor sportsman shops and get busy in your own kitchen making foods that are sure to please the hungry hikers in your life!

Crunchy Cake Sticks

After drying bread for bread crumbs, I decided to try drying cake for cake crumbs. I thought about using the crumbs as a topping on cakes or cupcakes or to build on them as a base for cheesecakes. When using them this way, you simply slice the cake into ½ inch slices, dry at 130 degrees for four to six hours and pulverize to a fine crumb.

As frequent campers though we got silly one night and made Crunchy Cake Sticks for an upcoming road trip. I have dried pound cake, yellow cake, chocolate cake, carrot cake and angel food cake. Before drying, I cut them up into sticks but any shape will do. I've considered slicing them ½ inch thick, cutting them again with cookie cutters and drying fun shapes for little people to enjoy. I'd also like to make a cream cheese dip to go along with our cake sticks but that didn't seem like a great idea for a fifteen-hour car ride.

You can make your cake at home or purchase one. The plan is to dry the cake without the frosting. If you buy something, make sure it is a pound cake or coffee cake without a sugary topping. I find it easier to make something at home unless you're short on time.

If you can make crunchy sticks from cake you can surely make them from breads too. I bake delicious loaves of sourdough bread and now not a piece will go to waste since they can be dried and used as bread sticks. Savory breads seasoned with my home-grown herbs will make perfect scoops when I'm enjoying spaghetti sauce. After growing the tomatoes and making rich gravy, I don't plan on missing one bite.

Store these crunchy sticks in an air-tight container. They are like little sponges just waiting to soak up any moisture in the air whatsoever.

Crunchy cake is definitely a conversation piece. It's nice to have something different to bring to a party….or a camping trip.

Proofing Bread

If you enjoy making bread at home, the dehydrator will be a pleasing addition to your baking routine. Sourdough is a favorite around our house and as soon as the weather begins to cool, I look forward to making bread.

My home is generally not as toasty warm as the dough would like on the chilly days when my mind turns to thoughts of bread, butter, and honey. So I'm left deciding where to put the dough so it will rise adequately.

Time to use the dehydrator! This technique works especially well if you can set the temperature. If you are able to remove the racks, make a space large enough for your bowl with room for the risen dough. Place the covered bowl into the dehydrator and set the temperature for 95 – 100 degrees. Let the dough sit for one to one and a half hours then continue with your recipe.

It is such a blessing to be able to let the dough proof without either having to heat the entire house or wait for hours as the bread rises to the desired level.

I'm always amazed at how many uses the dehydrator has available. Be sure to use it for more than just dried fruit!

Floral Fun

Flowers are so lovely and can be beautifully preserved by dehydrating. They work well in potpourris, flower arrangements, and wreaths.

I have a large bed of lavender that blooms and grows larger every year. I've found a lot of great uses for it. So much grows that it is hard to use in a timely fashion. If you have a flower like that, dry the flowers in your dehydrator and enjoy them year-round.

Small roses are very sweet to use when dried. Pick flowers from your garden to use in a tincture and once dried they'll be ready to use as long as you store them in an air-tight container.

Dried flower petals and colorful cardstock make very pretty stationary. Let a child try their hand at making pretty note cards to share with family members.

Carefully cut and clean the flowers. Dry them gently as you would herbs. Set your temperature at 100 degrees and dry for twelve to fourteen hours.

Storage

Since I've mentioned the step-by-step process of getting food into your home, let's consider storage methods. You'll acquire the foods you intend to dehydrate much as you do your ordinary groceries. Add to that work the process of all the steps you go through to dry foods. Washing, perhaps blanching, slicing or chopping, neatly loading trays and hours of patiently waiting. If you're not careful in the final step of storage, you'll essentially throw away hours of work (which began in the grocery, farmer's market or garden), your finances, hours of your precious time, and the whole reason you started this: food! A little moisture will lead to a lot of heartache. Mold ensues and suddenly you've got a new addition to the compost pile and suddenly Compost Heaven doesn't seem so heavenly after all.

Let your foods cool off before bagging them or sealing them in jars. The dehydrator gently heats the food as it dries. Putting warm food in an air-tight container creates condensation....the very element you were eliminating: water!

Add an oxygen packet then seal your containers after the food has cooled. Letting it cool on the tray is the best way to ensure you haven't added water to the storage container. Label the containers with contents and date and store in a cool location. Should you decide to dehydrate in quantity, put your food in labeled Mylar bags and store those bags in five or six gallon food-grade buckets. Make an inventory label for the bucket to keep track of what is coming and going from your stash. If you find you like the buckets, consider buying a screw-on lid. They're more expensive than snap-on lids but they make it much easier to access the foods if you need to get to them more frequently.

Have fun being creative with your new found skills. Only your imagination can hinder you now. My suggestion? Unleash it!

8 Stretching the Limits

Some days you just crave creativity. I had one of those days a few months ago. I'd recently read about putting meals together in canning jars. The ingredients were layered one upon another like a geological masterpiece. It occurred to me that the meal is not only convenient; it is also perfect for someone who dehydrates food.

You've probably already seen those jars full of cookie dough supplies with cute labels attached that tell the cook to add eggs and water. Everything is in one place except for the wet ingredients. This was the same except that the plan was for dinners instead of cookies.

As much as I love cookies (and that is my weakness if you must know), I really loved the idea of seeing meals stacked up in my basement. No longer wondering, "What's for dinner?" I'd be open to the options waiting in pretty little jars all in a row. And making these affords you the opportunity to buy what you need as the items go on sale. Convenience, best prices, ready-to-go dinner options....are you thinking what I'm thinking? How can we go wrong?

Meals as a Kit

If you decide to preserve meals as a kit (that's what I call them), you can begin the search for supplies you'll need on the internet. The choices are so numerous your head will be spinning. Plan to buy in bulk and make a lot of meals at a time. This is another great group project. If you have a canning-funnel, you'll put those quick dinners together in no time and with less mess.

That is what got my juices flowing. I noticed that a lot of food options were typical but not really what I wanted to use in my cooking. The whole point for me was to focus more on real food. Why would I add chemicals to my beautifully dehydrated foods?

One day I decided that instead of purchasing dried bean flakes for a Mexican dish, I'd just try drying my own. I started with a can of refried beans. I already knew how to make refried beans from scratch. The point wasn't learning how to do that but whether I liked the dried product I could create.

I'd decided if they were a hit, I'd make more by cooking the dried pinto beans next time.

I used a large can and gently spread the beans out on my non-stick sheet. Keeping them spread thin, I dried them for approximately six hours at 150 degrees. They were clearly dried when the tray of beans looked more like the floor of Death Valley than beans. They crumbled easily into a jar and were sealed up tight until I had time to test and taste them later. That large can of refried beans turned into a few ounces of dried beans. Already I was thinking camping food again.

It isn't always about convenience; sometimes it's about weight and portability. My mind began to stray from just a quick home-cooked meal to the tasty choices I'd soon have for a day hike or camp cook-stove. And what if I did the same thing with mashed potatoes to make my own potato flakes? For that matter, I could dry the beans or mashed potatoes and pulverize them as I did the sweet potatoes and pumpkins.

Naturally you won't need to do those things if you decide to purchase a large can of beans or potatoes online. Just crack open the seal and start layering. But if you're like me, you'll find you just can't help yourself.

So consider the possibilities. Look at the camping dinners in sealed Mylar bags next time you're in the camp section of a sporting-goods store. Notice what ingredients they list and think about what you can make yourself. Look through your cookbooks and decide what you'd like to try making for an easy dinner at home.

Remember that any variety of pasta, rice, lentils, or dried beans can be easily added to jars. Spices or dried herbs that you've harvested from your garden sit ready to add flavor and pizazz to meals. Imagine what a layer of sliced and dried tomatoes would look like. Or just add a layer of powdered tomatoes that will become a sauce at the point of cooking.

As you design the meal, keep track of how much dried food you're adding so you can determine how much water is needed to rehydrate the full meal. How much rice have you added? What amount of water do you normally use to cook that portion of rice? Same for potatoes or pasta. It isn't really rocket-science. And these suggestions aren't meant to frustrate you. You just need to become accustomed to looking at the ingredients as individuals and hydrate them accordingly.

When you're making a dish, always go lighter on the liquids since you can add more water, broth, or stock later. Before you know it, you've created something your family enjoys and asks for time and time again.

If you need a little boost, try what works for me. I often turn my kitchen into a cooking show (it never airs but what difference does it make if I'm having fun?). For a little more excitement, try out a new hair-do, play some Frank Sinatra, pull out a collection of your recently dehydrated foods and let the cooking begin! You're bound to have a great time, make a few duds and end up with a couple of outstanding recipes you'll become famous for. Cook with a little attitude and it will do wonders.

Cream of I Made it Myself Soup

We often think of using dehydrated foods when preparing the meal. Throw a little bit of potato or carrot into the soup or stew, add some green bell peppers or carrots to a pot of beans, or use dried fruits in a baked cobbler and you're making good use of your stash. But dehydrated foods are also good to use when making common ingredients used in some of the most basic recipes.

We're all familiar with the cream soups used in making a wide variety of dishes. Pull out a can of Cream of Whatever Soup and you're half-way to creating the "sauce" needed to hold dinner together. Really? What's in that can? And what if I can make something similar to it at home?

Let's do a dry run-through for a simple batch of Cream of La La Land Soup and then we'll dress the idea up a bit. Since it is easier to make larger batches and store them in a canning jar, we'll go for the jumbo size and you can split it down or supersize it later.

- 2 ½ c. instant non-fat dry milk
- ¾ c. cornstarch
- ¼ c. chicken or beef bouillon
- 2 T. dried onions
- 1 t. garlic powder
- ½ t. parsley
- ½ t. basil
- ½ t. thyme
- ½ t. black pepper
- ½ t. cayenne pepper (optional but I like it for the zip it adds)

The remaining ingredient is based on what you're making. Add 1/3 cup of finely chopped dehydrated mushrooms to make a full jar of Cream of Mushroom soup. If you'd prefer Cream of Celery soup, add 1/3 cup of dried celery. Cream of Broccoli is easily created using 1/3 cup of dried broccoli. You get the idea. If you want a richer bodied soup, increase the 1/3 cup of dried veggie to ½ cup. I generally want mine a little meatier…even if the meat is a mushroom in this case.

Mix all of the dry ingredients together and store in an air-tight container for up to one year. Before each use, shake the jar vigorously to mix and measure 1/3 cup of dry cream soup mix to 1 ¼ cup of water. Blend with a whisk and heat gently. Bring the soup to a boil and simmer for one minute to thicken. You have just made a perfectly suitable Cream of La La Land soup. Get busy and make a casserole or something. Show yourself to be strong and courageous in the kitchen….a mighty man or woman of great culinary skill, ready to stun the masses with your whisk and cast iron skillet.

Was that fun? Ready to try the dressed up version? You'll need a string of pearls or a bow tie. Time to look pretty. You don't really need them but it certainly seems like you should need some upscale duds.

Put together the same dried ingredients with the exception of the chicken or beef bouillon and rethink the herbs. Would your family prefer a different selection or are you serving this for a holiday meal? Consider sage, marjoram, rosemary, crumbled bay leaves, or chives.

I tend to like the earthy flavor the mushrooms add so I put them in any of the soups I design.

Store the ingredients in the air-tight container. You'll notice you're a little shy on the volume. That's alright since your beef or chicken bouillon flavor will be replaced with The Good Stuff. (The Good Stuff: anything of exceptional quality that you should be enjoying right now.) When you are ready to hydrate your soup, use ¾ cup of water and two to three ice cubes of your homemade chicken or beef stock to 1/3 cup of soup base. Heat to melt the ice cubes and continue cooking to a simmer as the soup thickens. Remove from the heat after one to two minutes of simmering and use as desired.

So that brings us to homemade stock. You should be making this periodically from beef bones (preferably grass-fed beef), chicken parts (neck, feet, wings, etc.) onions, celery, carrots, bay leaves, parsley, and thyme. You'll add solid nutrition provided by the marrow in the bones.

Put five pounds of chicken or beef bones into a pot with five quarts of water and a pinch of thyme, one bay leaf broken, an onion quartered or ½ cup of dried onion, two or three stalks of celery roughly chopped or ½ cup of dried celery, and one to two chopped carrots or 1/3 cup of dried carrots. Reduce heat and simmer for three hours, skimming the top as needed. As the stock cooks it will reduce and create a lovely base. Let it cool completely and strain into a large bowl. After it has cooled, I ladle it into ice trays (which are set aside for this purpose) and freeze. Once frozen, I place the cubes into large zip-lock bags and store them in the freezer. By having such small portions, it is very easy to use in daily cooking and adds taste and nutritional value that can't be beat!

Crackers and Other Crunchable Goodness

By now you should see the trend in dehydrating. Cut or prepare something thin, place it on a tray and dry it. If veggies and fruit work that way, shouldn't other things too?

Look through some cracker recipes and you'll find several options for dehydrating another treat in your kitchen. Use cooked steel-cut oats, flax seeds, whole-wheat flour, poppy seeds, sea salt, freshly ground pepper, grated cheese, herbs, spices, applesauce, nuts, or any other ingredient that strikes your fancy.

All you need do is prepare dough for crackers, spread it thinly on a non-stick sheet of parchment paper and dry at 130 degrees for six to eight hours. At this point the dough should be mostly dry but not completely. Lift the sheet of dough from the tray and place on a cutting board. With a pizza cutter, slice into approximately 1 ½ inch squares. Place back on the drying racks, this time with the moist side up and continue to dehydrate for another two or three hours until the crackers are crisp.

Pita breads and tortillas are great launching points for additional crunchy snacks. Sprinkled with any assortment of spices, they'll dry to a snappy finish if dried at 130 degrees for four to six hours. A brush of high-end extra virgin olive oil, a light handful of freshly grated parmesan cheese, and Italian spices makes a gourmet delicacy. Add some cayenne pepper for a little heat and let the party begin!

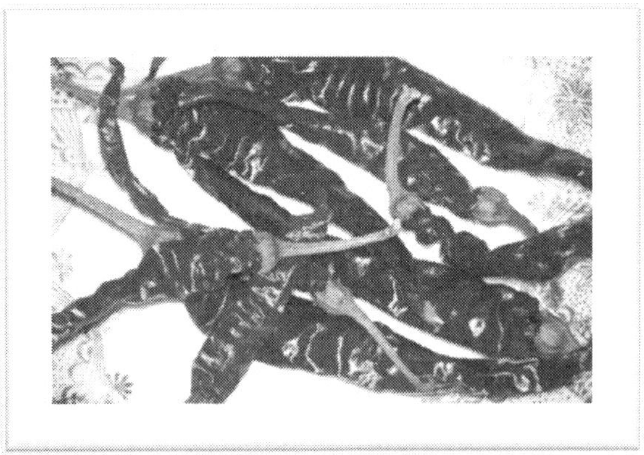

A Final Word

Whether you're dehydrating to save produce from your garden or to create a few easy to assemble meals in your kitchen, you've picked a very good choice for food preservation. Build your food store using frugal methods without increasing your demand for more electricity.

Begin a new routine of preserving foods the dehydrated way. You'll reap great benefits and feel good about your accomplishments. By having enough food for your family, you'll soon find yourself able to share. Being responsible with the food we have means throwing away less, saving more, and planning for the future wisely.

Now you know how to preserve just about any food you can imagine. So why not treat your family to The Good Stuff? Put the grocery store can down and pick up a canning jar full of flavor and nutrition using the ingredients you've dried yourself to create a product you can use that is easy to store, cheap on the old pocketbook, and just plain good.

Now you're ready to make something delicious, delightful and dehydrated!

Made in the USA
Monee, IL
04 November 2026

67378964R00058